A NEW DEAL FOR CHILDREN?

Re-forming education and care in England, Scotland and Sweden

Bronwen Cohen, Peter Moss, Pat Petrie and Jennifer Wallace

D1073808

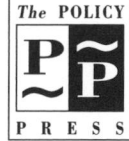

The POLICY
PRESS

First published in Great Britain in June 2004 by

The Policy Press
University of Bristol
Fourth Floor
Beacon House
Queen's Road
Bristol BS8 1QU
UK

Tel +44 (0)117 331 4054
Fax +44 (0)117 331 4093
e-mail tpp-info@bristol.ac.uk
www.policypress.org.uk

British Library Cataloguing in Publication Data
A catalogue record for this book is available from the British Library

Library of Congress Cataloging-in-Publication Data
A catalog record for this book has been requested

ISBN 1 86134 528 3 paperback

Bronwen Cohen is Chief Executive of Children in Scotland, Edinburgh, and a Visiting Professor at the Thomas Coram Research Unit, Institute of Education, University of London. **Peter Moss** is Professor of Early Childhood Provision, Thomas Coram Research Unit, Institute of Education, University of London. **Pat Petrie** is Professor of Education, Thomas Coram Research Unit, Institute of Education, University of London. **Jennifer Wallace** is Research Officer at Children in Scotland, Edinburgh.

The rights of Bronwen Cohen, Peter Moss, Pat Petrie and Jennifer Wallace to be identified as authors of this work have been asserted by them in accordance with the 1988 Copyright, Designs and Patents Act.

Cover design by Qube Design Associates, Bristol.
Front cover: photograph supplied by kind permission of www.third-avenue.co.uk
Printed and bound in Great Britain by Hobbs the Printers Ltd, Southampton.

Contents

Acknowledgements

This book is based on a research study funded by the UK Economic and Social Research Council (R000239373) and we would like to acknowledge the financial support provided by the Council.

Many people helped us in undertaking the research. Lisbeth and Bjorn Flising from the University of Göteborg helped us plan, and also supported, our Swedish fieldwork. Helen Fraser, Linda Kinney and Rod Harrison (Scotland), Gillian Pugh and Collette Kelleher (England) and Lisbeth Flising and Bjorn Flising (Sweden) commented on our case study chapters – though the final versions that appear in this book are entirely our responsibility. Annabelle Stapleton from the Thomas Coram Research Unit and Joan Telfer from Children in Scotland provided efficient administrative support for the study.

We were assisted by the relevant government departments in all three countries. In particular, we would like to thank Roger Halliday (Children and Education Statistics, Scottish Executive), Gill Robinson (Her Majesty's Inspectorate of Education in Scotland) and Marjorie Browning. We are also particularly grateful to the Scottish Executive for its support for a symposium to discuss the research findings, held in September 2003 at the world heritage site of New Lanark in Scotland, home to Robert Owen, the pioneer of integrated services for young children. We appreciated the comments on our findings offered at that event. They have helped to inform our final draft.

Finally, we would like to acknowledge the help and cooperation we received from all those we interviewed, from ministers to practitioners. We were impressed by the patience and courtesy shown to us by all our interviewees in helping us understand the changes that have taken place.

List of abbreviations

CCTC	Childcare Tax Credit
CYPU	Children and Young People's Unit (England)
DCMS	Department of Culture, Media and Sport
DES	Department of Education and Science
DfES (formerly DfEE)	Department for Education and Skills (formerly Department for Education and Employment) (England)
DoH	Department of Health (England)
DWP	Department for Work and Pensions (UK)
ECEC	Early Childhood Education and Care
EU	European Union
EYDCP	Early Years Development and Childcare Partnerships (England and Scotland)
EYNTO	Early Years National Training Organisation (England and Scotland)
FS	Foundation Stage (England)
GCSE	General Certificate in Secondary Education
GDP	gross domestic product
GNP	gross national product
GP	general practitioner (doctor)
HMIE (formerly HMIS)	Her Majesty's Inspectorate of Education (formerly Her Majesty's Inspectorate of Schools) (Scotland)
HNC	Higher National Certificate
HND	Higher National Diploma
LSAs	learning support assistants
LT Scotland	Learning and Teaching Scotland
MP	Member of Parliament
MSP	Member of the Scottish Parliament
NCS	New Community Schools (Scotland)
NOF	New Opportunities Fund (UK)
NTO	National Training Organisation (England and Scotland)
NVQ	National Vocational Qualification (England)
OECD	Organisation for Economic Co-operation and Development
Ofsted	Office for Standards in Education (England)
QCA	Qualifications and Curriculum Authority
SAT	Standard Assessment Tests (England)

SEED (formerly SOED)	Scottish Executive Education Department (formerly Scottish Office Education Department) (Scotland)
SEU	Social Exclusion Unit
SPRITO	National Training Organisation for Sport, Recreation and Allied Occupations (England and Scotland)
SSI	Social Services Inspectorate
SVQ	Scottish Vocational Qualification (Scotland)
UN	United Nations
UNCRC	United Nations Convention on the Rights of the Child
UNESCO	United Nations Educational, Scientific and Cultural Organisation
WFTC	Working Families Tax Credit

Glossary of terms

Barnskötare Childcare assistants in Sweden, who at one time would have trained in the upper secondary school (that is, when they were aged 16-19 years). Training is no longer available and the occupation is declining.

Breakfast clubs Services that provide care and breakfast for children in England and Scotland, often under the auspices of health promotion in areas of multiple deprivation.

Cabinet Office A department of the UK civil service that aims to support the government's delivery and reform programme.

Care Commission The Scottish Commission for the Regulation of Care (the Care Commission) is a national organisation set up in 2002 under the 2001 Regulation of Care (Scotland) Act to regulate and inspect Scottish care services including childcare and early years services.

Changing Children's Services Fund A UK-wide fund to encourage and develop integrated provision of children's services.

Child Benefit UK-wide universal benefit paid to parents of children under 16 (or under 19 in full-time education).

Childcare Tax Credit (CCTC) UK-wide tax credit providing funding to lower-income families for weekly childcare costs. Replaced in 2003-04 by the childcare element of the Working Tax Credit.

Childminders Registered workers in England and Scotland who look after other people's children in their own homes. Usually paid directly by parents/carers but may sometimes be employed by other agencies.

Children's Centres A small number of centres in England and to a lesser extent in Scotland that in general seek to provide integrated services for pre-school children and their families encompassing education, care and other provision. In England a target has been set to establish 1,000 children's centres in disadvantaged areas by 2008.

Children's trusts Currently being established in England, bringing together a range of agencies including social services, health and education to jointly plan, commission, finance and sometimes deliver services. Most areas should have trusts by 2006.

Classroom assistant School worker in England and Scotland, supporting teachers in the classroom.

Commune Local government area in Sweden.

Comprehensive Spending Review Conducted by the UK Treasury to determine spending and outcomes for government departments over a three-year period.

Connexions Service Multi-agency information, advice and guidance service in England.

Day nurseries Centre-based services in England and Scotland, with full-day provision for children under five years old.

Devolution The process by which Scotland regained its Parliament and Wales gained its Assembly in 1999.

Early Excellence Centres Centres designated as part of a programme in England intended to develop, demonstrate and broadcast models of delivery of centre-based, integrated multi-agency services for children, families and the wider community. Superseded by *Children's Centres.*

Familjedaghem Swedish family daycare or 'childminders' who, in Sweden, are employed by the *commune.*

Family Centres UK centres providing childcare, early education and family support services.

Förskola Swedish pre-school centres for children from one to six years old.

Förskoleklass Swedish pre-school class for six-year-old children.

Förskollare Swedish pre-school teacher.

Fritidshem Swedish free-time services, or school-age childcare services.

Fritispedagogue Swedish free-time pedagogue, a worker who works in free-time care services.

Grundskola Swedish compulsory schooling.

Gymnasie skola (Gymnasium) Swedish upper secondary school for young people aged 16-19.

Her Majesty's Inspectorate of Education (HMIE) Scottish agency that inspects education provision.

HM Treasury The UK civil service department responsible for formulating and putting into effect the government's financial and economic policy, headed by the Chancellor of the Exchequer.

Housing Benefit UK-wide benefit contributing to housing costs.

Income Support UK-wide benefit supplementing income of those on low incomes.

Kurator Swedish school-based social worker or counsellor.

Lärarförbundet Swedish teachers' union.

Learning and Teaching Scotland (LT Scotland) Scottish national body (funded by SEED) covering all matters relating to the curriculum in the pre-school, primary and secondary education sectors in Scotland. LT Scotland is required to advise the Scottish Executive on any aspect of the learning experiences of children and young people up to the age of 18, and on any issue that may have an effect on those learning experiences. It also provides guidance and support on the curriculum for schools, local education authorities and others.

Local authority Local government in the UK.

Ministry for Social Welfare Swedish civil service department responsible for care and welfare services.

Municipality Swedish local government area.

Neighbourhood nurseries English initiative to develop centre-based services for children in disadvantaged areas.

New Community Schools (NCS) Scottish initiative to integrate children's services within a school setting.

New Deal A key part of the UK government's strategy to get people back to work. It aims to give people on benefits the help and support they need to look for work, including training and job preparation.

Nursery classes Classes in primary schools in England and Scotland providing mainly part-time education for three- and four-year-olds.

Nursery schools Schools in England and Scotland dedicated to providing education for three- and four-year-olds.

Nursery vouchers UK-wide scheme in the mid-1990s to develop pre-school provision by giving parents vouchers to be exchanged for services for their children. Introduced only on pilot basis and scrapped in 1997.

Out-of-school care Care for schoolchildren outside school hours and during holidays. For the most part aimed at working parents.

Parental leave Entitlement to leave from work to care for a young child, available equally to mothers and fathers.

Pedagogy A term that in continental Europe refers to the support of children's overall development and their education in the widest sense of that word.

Play groups Centre-based services in England and Scotland providing mainly part-time provision for two- to four-year-olds, usually run by non-profit private groups.

Pre-school services Services provided to children before they reach compulsory school age.

Primary school Initial compulsory education in the UK.

Public–private partnership Joint funding of services and initiatives from both private and public funds (such as the Scottish school-building programme).

Pump-priming funds Short-term funding for start-up costs of services, common in UK policy.

Rektor A general Swedish term, the equivalent of director, that can be used across many educational settings. In this book it refers to school principals, including those who head a cluster of schools.

School-age childcare Childcare provided to children of school age out of school hours.

Scottish Executive Scottish devolved government. The Executive is led by a First Minister who is nominated by the Parliament and in turn appoints the other Scottish ministers who make up the Cabinet.

Scottish Office Pre-devolution civil service department responsible for Scottish policies including education and care.

Scottish Parliament Seat of Scottish government in respect of devolved areas.

Secondary school Compulsory and post-compulsory schooling within the UK for children who have progressed through primary school (usually moving to secondary school at the age of 12).

Skolverket Swedish National Agency for Education.

Social Exclusion Unit (SEU) The UK SEU aims to coordinate work on social exclusion across government departments.

Social Inclusion Unit The Scottish civil service unit charged with developing and promoting social justice policy throughout the Executive.

Social Services Inspectorate (SSI) The SSI is part of the UK central government Department of Health, providing professional advice on social services matters to government, inspections of local authority social services departments and assessments of their performance.

Statutory maternity leave The length of time a mother can take off work before and after the birth of a child, as decreed by government.

Sure Start UK initiative to provide support services for young children in disadvantaged areas.

Targeted services Service available only to those who meet certain criteria.

Tax credits A system of payments to individuals made through the UK Inland Revenue and linked to employment rather than the benefits system.

Universal services Services offered to all members of a society.

Welsh Assembly Seat of Welsh government in respect of devolved areas.

Westminster government Seat of English government and 'reserved' UK matters.

Whitehall English civil service, based in London and responsible for 'reserved' areas of policy.

Working Families Tax Credit (WFTC) UK-wide tax credit for families – either couples or lone parents – if they: have one or more children living with them; work at least 16 hours per week (for couples, both must be working 16 hours unless one partner is incapacitated); and have savings of no more than £8,000. Replaced by Working Tax Credit 2003-04.

Part One:
International comparisons of social and educational reforms: background and contexts

ONE

Introduction

A new deal for children? is about how the national governments in three countries – England, Scotland and Sweden – have changed the relationship between three types of children's services: *early childhood education and care* (services that go under names such as pre-schools, kindergartens, nurseries and nursery classes, all for children below compulsory school age); *schools* (for children of compulsory school age and beyond); and *school-age childcare* (services that, among other functions, provide for the children of working parents before school starts in the morning, at the end of the school day and during holidays). At around the same time, in the mid- to late 1990s, each country brought responsibility for all of these services together in the same government department: education. This book arises from the authors' research into these reorganisations and other related reforms. The reforms that we have studied raise important practical, political and theoretical issues: about the meaning of and relationship between children's education and care; about the relationship between these areas, family life and employment; about the work of those engaged face to face with children; and, not least, about how these changes affect, and are affected by, children's relationship to society and society's understanding of childhood.

We need to recognise that the three countries in our study do not have the same national status. England and Scotland form part of one state, the United Kingdom (UK), while Sweden is a unitary nation state. England and Scotland, however, are distinct countries and may justifiably be treated separately from each other. Even after the Treaty of Union in 1707, which ended the separate Scottish Parliament, Scotland had its own legislation and distinct legal and educational systems. With devolution in 1999, Scotland has regained its parliament, is governed by a Scottish Executive, and has legislative, executive and financial responsibility for the services discussed in this book. Although Scotland is much more similar to England than to Sweden in most respects, there are nevertheless important and growing differences between the two countries, and since devolution Scotland has enjoyed substantial freedom to develop its own policy, provision and practice. The main limitations on this independence are the responsibility that continues to rest with the UK government in a number of relevant areas and the growing influence of HM Treasury on many aspects of policy. We discuss these issues in later chapters.

This introductory chapter provides a background to the study. It then provides a brief outline of how the study was accomplished, together with some reflections on comparative research, including considerations on the English language and the implications of its increasing international dominance. Finally, there is a brief outline of the contents of the chapters and appendix that follow.

The reforms

Within the same short period of time, the governments of England, Scotland and Sweden each made a rather similar decision. Each government decided to place national responsibility for early childhood services, schools and school-age childcare – for policy, oversight, funding and administration – within its education department: Sweden in 1996, Scotland in 1997 and England in 1998. Some countries had already integrated responsibility for all early childhood services (childminding, day nurseries, kindergartens and so forth) within either welfare or education. For example, Nordic countries had located them within welfare, and New Zealand and Spain within education (although in Spain a law passed at the end of 2002 will, if implemented, remove children aged up to three years out of education again, and make early childhood once again a separate departmental responsibility). No other countries, as far as we were aware at the time had brought together all early childhood services, schools *and* school-age childcare services within national departments of education.

We say England, Scotland and Sweden made a 'rather' similar decision because, as we will show, national contexts have affected the history, implementation and meaning of these processes of departmental reorganisation. We will see, for example, how the three countries have different approaches to the welfare state, understandings of children and childhood, training for work with children and the powers and the responsibilities of local communities compared with those of central government. We will also find that these factors are interrelated.

We concentrate on the relationships between three services – early childhood education and care, schools and school-age childcare – prior to departmental reorganisation, how it is today and what it might become. These services are mass providers: they are intended for children's daily use; they are either already universal in coverage or are becoming increasingly widely used; and their ongoing expansion is a matter of public policy. In all three countries, some important but more targeted or occasional services for children – primarily health services – remained outside education at the time of departmental integration. We have paid attention to the relationship between services inside and outside education, as well as noting the subsequent transfer of some of these services (such as child welfare) into education – in Scotland in 1999 and in England in 2003. In these cases, education, which already has responsibility for many major services, seems to exercise an inexorable gravitational pull. This has not happened in Sweden, but in that country there is a strong relationship between services now in education and leave policies to support employed parents, and we consider that relationship too.

The processes we examine raise many important issues about practice within provision for children. But they also raise macro issues. In particular, the changes we shall document need to be viewed in relation to their potential consequences for three important areas. First, these organisational changes may affect *the childhoods lived by children*, including the ways in which social control is exercised. Second, the changed relationships between the three sets of services may affect their relative status and *the balance of power* between them. Third, and closely related to the last point, is the issue of whether departmental reforms in relationships between services lead to more extensive *integration or coordination* of services, including the emergence of new institutions with their accompanying occupations and professions, or closer collaboration between existing institutions and occupations.

Children's childhoods and social control

The economies of the three countries on which the book focuses are post-industrial; they have developed from earlier agricultural and industrial bases into more predominantly service economies and, with the development of new technologies, knowledge-based economies. They are countries with high levels of female and male employment, and need a flexible and educated workforce, capable of adapting to the new requirements of evolving employment. The services that are the central subject of this book form an essential part of the social and economic infrastructure of each country. They become an everyday part of the lives of the great majority of families and, with health services, form the backbone of social provision for children and their parents, and, some would argue, are not only a necessary resource but also a locus of social control.

The position of the oldest and most powerful of these services, the school, is well established. In the Minority World of (post-) industrial countries especially, a society without universal schooling has long been almost impossible to imagine – although less than 200 years ago it was the norm. We are passing through a period when childhood is increasingly institutionalised, collectivised and brought into the public sphere. Over the past century, the number of years that children spend in school has increased, higher education has been developed and hugely expanded, and 'lifelong learning' has become a familiar government aim. The population, especially children and young people, has increasingly been institutionalised by education.

The institutionalisation of childhood does not stop with the school, however. The number of children under the age of 12 years using so-called childcare services has expanded. In post-industrial countries, early childhood education and care and school-age childcare services have become increasingly demanded and used – whether to free parents for participation in the workforce or to begin the processes of education at a younger life stage. From being somewhat reluctantly used by a minority of parents, these services have increasingly become a community resource valued by the majority. In Sweden, for example:

> ... enrolling children from age one in full-day pre-schools has become generally acceptable. What was once viewed as either a privilege of the wealthy for a few hours a day, or an institution for needy children and single mothers, has become, after 70 years of political vision and policy making, an

> unquestionable right of children and families. (Lenz Taguchi and
> Munkammer, 2003, p 27)

Sweden may be (along with its Nordic neighbour Denmark) a world leader in
providing universal access to high-standard services, but it is plausible that a
similar trend to general acceptance and use of such services will follow in most
countries.

These processes of institutionalisation have enormous consequences for the
childhoods lived by children, including children's use of time and space, the
activities they undertake, the peer groups with which they interact, and the
types and levels of surveillance and control to which they are subjected. For
example, children and young people have been increasingly subjected to control
exercised through educational establishments, as the control that was once
predominantly exercised through the family and through employment has
waned. The institutionalisation arising from the spread of education and care
services is not necessarily a retrograde step. Rather, it involves both possibilities
and risks, which are themselves affected by the movement towards more
integration or coordination between services. Closer relations between services
and professionals can bring benefits, such as greater continuity and security for
children and parents, but they can also make it easier to govern the child
through more effective surveillance and control.

New relationships and the balance of power

Questions of power also arise in the relationship of institutions with each
other. In later chapters of this book, we shall see that the institution of the
school emerges as particularly powerful. Closer relations between the school
and other services can result in what some in Sweden refer to as 'schoolification':
the increasing power of the school in the lives of children and families,
accompanied by the dominance of school professionals and school culture. Yet
new relationships may lead to something very different: the creation of a meeting
place where different institutions seek to build relationships of equality, in
which no one institution dominates and all strive to work together with new,
shared understandings. Put another way, closer relationships may be stimulating,
opening up new experiences for all; but they may also be stifling if one partner
tries to dominate what are seen as more vulnerable institutions.

The school is often seen as a purely educational establishment. But there
have always been instances of schools seeking to provide services beyond
children's education. Interest has revived in recent years in schools building on
their comprehensive presence and universal availability and extending their
services to their local communities. This was particularly apparent in the United
States (US) in the 1990s:

> [Here] a new and unprecedented wave of school–community initiatives has
> appeared over the last decade and grown exponentially (Kagan, 1997;

Melaville and Blank, 1999). As 'schools have become the location of choice for collaborative programmes' (Wang, et al, 1998, p 3), there is widespread development of school-linked health and human service programmes.... They have various titles: school-linked services, community schools, extended-services schools or full-service (community) schools. (Moss et al, 1999, p 18)

The recent Organisation for Economic Co-operation and Development (OECD) study of early childhood education and care (ECEC) also suggests that relations are changing between early childhood services and compulsory schooling, and concludes that there "is a welcome trend towards increased cooperation between ECEC and the school system in terms of both policy and practice". Two reasons for this are suggested. First, increased attention paid to children's transitions from early childhood services to schools "has led to a greater policy focus on building bridges across administrative departments, staff training, regulations and curricula". Second, the increasing policy stress on lifelong learning has led to recognition of the need for closer cooperation and coherence, recognising "early childhood – from birth to 8 – as an important phase for developing important dispositions and attitudes toward learning" (OECD, 2001, p 128).

However, the OECD report also sounds a warning note, one that recurs throughout this book, and reminds us that most relationships entail taking the rough with the smooth. Closer relationships, whether through more coordination or complete integration between separate services, may carry risks as well as offering opportunities:

> The needs of young children are wide, however, and there is a risk that increased co-operation between schools and ECEC could lead to a school-like approach to the organisation of early childhood provision. Downward pressure on ECEC to adopt the content and methods of the primary school has a detrimental effect on young children's learning. Therefore, it is important that early childhood is viewed not only as a preparation for the next stage of education (or even adulthood), but also as a distinctive period where children live out their lives. Stronger co-operation with schools is a positive development as long as the specific character and traditions of quality early childhood practice are preserved. (OECD, 2001, p 129)

Questions of integration

Many of the people interviewed in the course of our research used the term 'integration'. It is also found in many policy documents. Usually integration is seen as a positive aim for children's services, but its meaning is sometimes problematic. Relationships between children's services and policy sectors have been complicated in the past because, as this institutional landscape of childhood has formed, large fissures have appeared. In the period of childhood before compulsory education, provision in most countries has been split between 'childcare services', designed primarily to enable parents to remain in or to re-enter the labour market, and nursery or early years education services, whose main purpose has been children's learning. With school-age children, a similar split has become apparent among childcare, play and education services, as 'school-age childcare services' have emerged and developed at a later stage in national histories than childcare for young children (Petrie, 1994; OECD, 2001, p 53). A divide has also existed between pre-school services and compulsory schooling, although some early childhood services have been provided in schools within the education system, and it has long been believed that one purpose of *pre-school services* is to prepare children for compulsory schooling. The relationship between *childcare services* (such as childminders and day nurseries) and later schooling has been distant. More generally, the 'early childhood' field as a whole – practitioners, policy makers, trainers and researchers – has generally kept itself to itself.

In recent years, some bridging of these divides has been contemplated and even begun. In the early childhood, if not the compulsory school, field, discourse has been growing about the closeness of the relationship between education and care. To cite three examples: the 1992 European Council of Ministers Recommendation on Child Care refers to the need for childcare services to combine 'reliable care' (a service for parents) with a 'pedagogical approach' (practice that supports the child's physical, emotional, social and intellectual development); in 1998, the document that provides the foundation of the government's Childcare Strategy in England asserts that "there is no sensible distinction between good early education and care" (DfEE, 1998, para 1.4), implying that the processes and values of one are subsumed in the other; lastly, a recent cross-national review of policies for young children and their families defined its theme as "early childhood education *and* care" (OECD, 2001; emphasis added), with the clear understanding that the two areas could not sensibly be separated.

For all three countries, the initial reform of departmental responsibilities concentrated many children's services within a single area of government, thus removing one potential obstacle to forming new relationships between the three sets of services. However, it may be misleading to think of such administrative reforms as necessarily *integrating* services.

'Integrate' can be a beguiling word. It is frequently used in British policy documents but is less often defined. Consequently, the meaning is often unclear. A recent example of this is a Scottish Executive consultative document, *Integrated strategy for the early years*, which presents 'a coherent vision of integrated services which together can meet the universal, and more individual needs of families and young children' (Scottish Executive, 2003b, para 2). Yet the document uses a wide range of other terms about the relationship between services: 'align', 'a coordinated and coherent framework', 'joined up working', 'working well together', 'joint planning, commissioning and single system, service delivery', 'a single service', 'complementary role' and 'an integrated approach'. What is unclear is whether these are all considered synonymous with 'integrated' or indicate subtle shades of meaning about future relations between services.

Even in the substantial academic literature on the concept of integration in various policy fields, the relationship between 'integration' and other concepts, such as 'coordination', is not clear. The US National Center for Service Integration, established in 1991, defined 'service integration' as a "process by which a range of educational, health and social services are delivered in a coordinated manner to improve outcomes for children and families" (Ryan, 2003, p 36). In the field of social services, several authors have proposed a 'continuum of integration', starting with a minimal level of information sharing or awareness raising, then moving through various stages such as 'communication', 'cooperation' and 'collaboration' to full 'integration' or 'fusion' (Konrad, 1996; Ryan et al, 2002).

Specifically in the field of ECEC, and with a particular focus on decision making, Bradley (1982, pp 32-4) distinguishes 'eight aspects of coordination'. These ranged from 'dissociation' ("where sectors take a positive decision not to work with others"), through 'cooperation' ("working together towards a common end") and 'federation' ("separate sectors working together [with] each accepting the other's goal"), to 'unification' ("where services have a single administration"). However, Bradley notes that services administered by one department "has not necessarily produced a unified service".

In this book, we define 'service integration' as the extent to which services are merged or fused across a number of dimensions, both structural and conceptual. Structural dimensions include departmental responsibility, staffing, funding and regulation. Conceptual dimensions include principles, values, identity, approaches to practice, understandings of children and of learning, care and other purposes. Services, therefore, can vary from being totally integrated, as when previously separate services merge to become one, to being very partially integrated, as when, for example, they are the responsibility of one department and covered by the same regulatory regime but with little other signs of integration. Indeed, like Bradley, we would argue that being in the same department is not by itself enough to make services 'integrated'.

We would distinguish 'integration' from other concepts expressing closer relations between services. Services can be subject to measures that are intended to provide for closer and more effective working but fall short of integration. In these cases, perhaps, terms implying a more complementary approach between separate and distinct services, such as 'joined-up' working, coordination or collaboration, would be more appropriate and less misleading. Also, services may be partially integrated, for example by coming within the same departmental responsibility and regulatory framework, but remain distinct and therefore subject to efforts to promote closer working relations.

The study

The research on which this book is based was carried out between 2000 and 2002. We briefly outline in this section the research questions and methodology and offer a few reflections on cross-national research, especially linguistic considerations and issues of power.

The research began with a number of questions. What was the history of this move to departmental integration? What had preceded it and influenced it, and why was it done? How was the process carried out? How far beyond departmental reorganisation did the integration process extend? Was departmental integration accompanied by changes in staffing, funding and access, management and organisation of services, content and practice? What conditions supported or inhibited the integration process? At this early stage, were any consequences of the reform process discernible?

While our attention was mainly on the three services brought together within education departments, we were also aware of the many other services for children and families, mostly remaining outside education. What was the relationship between the three 'education-based' services and these other services? How did departmental integration affect this relationship? Taking a broad view, what is the new landscape of children's services that is emerging from new relationships and divisions of responsibility?

In seeking answers to these questions, and interpreting the differences we observed between countries, we have paid particular attention to national contexts. We have tried better to understand these contexts so as to make better sense of the policy and service developments that we were observing. From the beginning, we identified four aspects as particularly important: welfare regimes, social conditions (in particular employment, poverty and diversity), the relationship between national and local government, and the rather more intangible issue of understandings of childhood and the relationship between care and education. We were also aware of the very different histories of services in the three countries, histories that had produced very different services by the late 1990s, in particular when we compared Sweden with England and Scotland.

The research

Details of the research are presented in the Appendix. To summarise, in each of the three countries we worked at two levels, national and local. Nationally, we conducted interviews with key informants from government departments and various national organisations (public agencies, trade unions, voluntary organisations, and so on), as well as with a number of researchers and other individual experts. Altogether, we interviewed 72 informants at this national level.

Then in each country three local authorities were visited (referred to below as 'study local authorities'). In each local authority we visited a range of services: at least one centre for young children, one school-age childcare service, one primary school and one secondary school, and sometimes more. These authorities were selected in consultation with national-level informants, with the intention that at least two in each country should be considered to be successfully implementing reforms and at least one local authority should have a record of departmental integration pre-1996-98. At least one local authority per country contained a large rural area.

Overall, we visited nine local authorities. In each authority we interviewed between eight and 12 informants, working in specific services or at local authority level. We also visited a range of services: in each area at least one nursery, one free-time service, one primary school and one secondary school, and sometimes more.

These interviews and visits were supplemented with a wide range of national and local documents, many of which were identified by interviewees as 'key documents'.

Conducting cross-national research

Many different perspectives and experiences contributed to the study. But we would like to comment especially on some aspects of the way we first understand and subsequently represent these perspectives and experiences in conducting and reporting cross-national research. In doing so, we are very likely to raise more questions than we can answer; nevertheless, we think the exercise is worthwhile for the sake of transparency and to remind ourselves and our readers of the power of language and of some of the problems inherent in translation.

In conducting the research, we set out to understand and represent the perspectives of our various informants and to draw on national documentation so as to construct three national case studies, which form the core of the book. It is a truism that the processes of research are affected by the identities and perspectives of those who conduct it. While as members of a research team we are in many ways different from one another as well as from our informants, we do not intend to dwell on considerations of gender, age, profession or academic discipline, enticing though such an exploration might be. However, because we are reporting a cross-national study, we would like to offer some brief reflections on differences between ourselves, and between us and our informants, arising out of nationality and, related to this, differences of language.

Two of the authors of this book live and work in England and two in Scotland, but none in Sweden. We have taken several measures to try to compensate, as best we can, for this lack of a Swedish perspective. Over the years we have visited Sweden frequently, and have collaborated with a number of Swedish researchers. We came to the study with some prior knowledge of policy and provision, and some of the related debates, in Sweden. Our extensive interviews in Sweden for the study described in this book extended our knowledge. Some of the key documents from Sweden were already translated into English, and we had some others translated for us. We were also assisted by two Swedish consultants, who provided background information, helped us to arrange interviews, and commented on what we had written about Sweden.

None of these measures, however, makes up for the absence of a Swedish researcher working on an equal basis across the whole study: our best efforts fail to compensate for the absence of a distinctly Swedish perspective contributing to the study's design and analysis. Without a Swedish partner, it is all too easy to miss nuanced but important aspects of children's services in Sweden: deep-seated assumptions that may be taken for granted by Swedish informants but overlooked by non-Swedish researchers, concepts that lose meaning when translated into English, historical and cultural influences on reform that are not obvious to outsiders. In particular, it is difficult for outsiders to achieve a deep understanding of the history of service developments in Sweden, including debates about the relationship between 'childcare' and education, pre-schools and schools.

Moreover, the absence of a Swedish partner deprived us of an external perspective on England or Scotland. One of the values of cross-national work is that it can articulate a wide range of assumptions, taken-for-granted practices and tacit understandings – especially when observers from other countries bring their perspectives to the study. For instance, examining English or Scottish policies, services and practices through Swedish eyes would inevitably lead to challenging and critical questions. Why do you do that? Why are things organised that way? What is the thinking behind that? Why do you call it that? To extend the optical metaphor, a 'Swedish lens' would also have made it easier for us to discern the really important issues, especially when confronted (as has been the case in England and Scotland since 1997) by a blizzard of policy statements, initiatives, guidelines, targets and other documents.

A final point concerns language. Language is not only a means of communication: it is also the way in which we construct meaning and therefore our understandings of the world, ourselves and others. Often cross-national work involves countries with different native languages. Especially if researchers are not multilingual, they are faced with the problem of how to gain understandings of their subject of study in another country without being able to use the tool of language with which that subject is constructed.

Many Swedes speak excellent English, and we were often accompanied on local visits by Swedes who could help with interpretation. But the dynamic is quite different from speaking with someone in his or her native language. Indeed, the excellent English of many Swedes may lull the visiting Briton into a false sense of confidence: it is easy to forget that the person speaking such good English, especially in using technical terms, may be involved in some difficult decisions and approximations. While translation cannot be avoided, whether of conversation or of documents, it is invariably problematic. In particular, concepts and terms that have a very precise meaning in one country and language can easily lose that precision in translation: the 'otherness' of the concept or term is lost as it is grasped and forced to fit into another language.

A classic example of this is the concept of 'pedagogy'. We shall discuss the concept in Chapter Two, but for the moment suffice it to say that 'pedagogy' involves theories and practices premised upon a holistic approach to working with children and the inseparability of learning, care and, more generally, upbringing at the level of daily work. The concept is widely understood in continental Europe but not in the English-speaking world.

This situation of ignorance is perpetuated since 'pedagogy' is often translated into English as 'education', while 'pedagogue' (a member of the profession working with 'pedagogy') often ends up as 'teacher' or 'educator'. In this way, a concept that is important in Sweden and many other countries has been rendered virtually absent from the English language. Nor does the term 'childcare' capture the services and practices that would often be referred to as 'pedagogical' in Sweden. For 'childcare' has gained a common usage in the English language that is far narrower than 'pedagogy'. When the public, press or politicians talk of 'childcare' they envisage the provision of safe physical care for children with employed parents: practitioners may, of course, have a wider concept in mind when they use 'childcare', but this is a minority view. References to 'childcare' in the book do not, therefore, assume that the term is self-evident or neutral in its meaning – but then no terms are.

Behind the practical problems of translation, there is an important issue of power. As English becomes ever more dominant as a world language (not least in the policy and research fields covered by this book), there is a growing risk of losing diversity. Important concepts and terms from a variety of cultural and linguistic contexts become endangered species, overwhelmed by English-language concepts and terms that are the product of a very specific political, social and cultural context. Important research and work on practice that is not translated into English is ignored: for example, it does not appear in literature databases and, therefore, in literature reviews. The dominance of English extends even to English-Scottish linguistic and policy relations. Scottish English is not identical to that spoken in England, including the English of the Westminster government. Indeed, the closeness of Scottish English and English English can itself obscure differences in meaning. The power of Westminster English is compounded by the dominance of those areas of Westminster policy that apply to UK-wide provisions (such as tax credits, parental leave or Sure Start – a HM Treasury initiated targeted initiative in a devolved policy area for children under the age of four living in disadvantaged areas, discussed in Chapter Three). Such initiatives and the language in which they are couched contribute to the shape, language and conceptualisation of early years services in Scotland.

Native speakers of the dominant language rarely see the problem, as they are immune from having to translate their work into other languages and do not have to struggle with translating work in other languages into English. Those who are not native English speakers are often either too polite to confront the issue or can see little point in doing so, accepting the inevitability of the increasing use of English. We do not exempt ourselves from this criticism of the hegemony of English and of the failure of many native English speakers to recognise and address the issues of understanding and power that follow.

In this book, we introduce the main Swedish services and occupations working in those services in Chapter Five. In each case, we give the name in Swedish and provide a literal English translation that we use subsequently. For example, we use the English term 'pre-school' to translate *förskola*, the main Swedish early childhood service, preferring this literal translation to 'nursery', a term frequently used for early childhood centres in England and Scotland and also for nursery education in Scotland. In so doing, we realise that 'pre-school' is itself problematic. Some people object to its usage because it seems to define early years services, their users and staff, in terms of the school; it may also connect with ideas of earlier stages of education as merely a preparation for what follows. Nevertheless, we use 'pre-school' because it is a direct translation of *förskola* and because it can be seen as expressing the chronological relationship between the two services rather than suggesting any subordination of the earlier stage.

This approach only scratches the surface of the larger issue of linguistic dominance. But it may serve to remind the reader that the issue exists and that language carries important cultural and social meanings. (The reader may like to consider the different associations and images generated by the terms 'pre-school' and 'nursery' or by another set of contrasting terms – 'free-time services' and 'school-age childcare' – to illustrate the role of language in reflecting and reproducing meaning.)

When we want to refer to services in general, encompassing all three countries, rather than to the services of a particular country, we have adopted three generic terms: **early childhood services** for services for children below compulsory school age; **school-age childcare services** for services providing play, informal learning activities and care for children attending school; and **school** for services providing formal learning for children of compulsory school age.

The rest of the book

The book comprises three parts. This first part continues with Chapter Two, in which we examine and compare some important aspects of national context in our three countries in order to provide the reader with some means of making sense of the subsequent discussion of the reform process. Part Two consists of three national case studies, each describing the reform process and related issues. Before discussing the policies of our three countries in depth, we look at three imaginary children, and their usual school or pre-school days and educational and childcare histories. The intention is to begin each chapter with some concrete examples to highlight the main ways in which national policy plays out at local level. Although the children are fictitious, in describing their experience we are drawing on the many visits we have made to childcare and educational institutions in the course of this and other research. The children live in England, Scotland and Sweden, countries that have all undergone recent reforms bringing childcare, early years education and the school into the same administrative system. The extent and manner of the reforms is distinctive in each country, although Scotland and England have much in common. But, even before departmental reorganisation, there were other substantial differences in policy, provision and practice between the three countries.

The final section makes overall comparisons between the three countries and considers further developments. Chapter Six switches from a country focus to a thematic focus, looking cross-nationally at the extent and nature of structural and conceptual integration. We also try to make a broad assessment of the reform process in each country and the influences that have shaped it. What has it been about and why has it taken its particular course? In conclusion, Chapter Seven considers possible future directions both for the 'education-based' services and for their relations to other children's services. Looking forward, what are the risks and what are the opportunities in the developments we describe? To what extent is further integration called for and what forms might it take? How else might relationships be reconfigured?

Our research ended in 2002, but the world has gone on. There have been further policy developments, especially in England and Scotland where, since the change of government in 1997, a continuous process of change has been under way, sometimes bordering on the frenetic. In writing this book, we have tried to take account of the most recent developments that have occurred since the study ended – although, necessarily, without the benefit of obtaining our informants' perspectives on them. Our research, therefore, is a snapshot of work in progress, not a formal record of a finished product.

Note

In the text, where pounds sterling, the currency for England and Scotland, have been converted into euros, the exchange rate is £1 = €1.43. Swedish kroner (SEK) have been converted into euros at the rate of SEK1 = €0.108. These rates applied on 14 August 2003.

TWO

Contexts

Before examining the reform process in each of our three countries, we examine here the different contexts in which these changes have taken place. Policies and institutions do not drop out of the sky; to some extent they are formed and reformed, in part at least, by structural conditions: the evolving social and political features that characterise a given society. Structural conditions provide the national, macro-level contexts for reforms, and vary over time and between countries.

In this chapter we analyse four broad contextual dimensions: the people and the economy; welfare regimes; government; and understandings of children. We have tried, where possible, to treat England and Scotland separately, though in some cases separate information is not available. The importance of the contextual dimensions will become apparent when we turn, in the following chapters, to consider the reform process and why it took the course it did in each country. Apart from contributing to the interpretation of national processes of reform and to understandings of cross-national similarities and differences, such contextual analyses caution against over-simplified ideas about the possibility of transferring policy and practice from one country to another. Without the right contextual conditions, policies do not travel well – indeed they may not be able to travel at all.

Enduring structural characteristics provide a context that helps to explain long-term continuities in national policies, spanning even periods of government by different political parties. Policy formation is not just a matter of assembling evidence and inferring from it what works, nor are policies influenced only by vested interests and other party political considerations. They are also a matter of mindsets, habitual ways of constructing problems and determining how to respond to them, understandings of the world that make certain courses of action seem self-evidently correct, and others unthinkable and unrealistic. And such mindsets are constructed within and through the influence of national contexts, structural forces whose capacity to govern our thoughts and actions must be recognised if we are to understand the societies in which we live. There may be a risk from this line of argument of overstating the power of context, seemingly allowing no space for agency and inducing a resignation as damaging as the naivety that flows from ignoring structure. Yet recognition of the significance of context does not justify the over-determined view that radical change is not possible in a country because its context is immutable. The exercise of social agency in the field of social policy requires social understanding that can proceed from contextual structures being made visible and available for reflection. Contexts themselves are not immutable: countries can, and sometimes do, make substantial policy shifts. There is always room for agency, all the more so when it is informed by an understanding of context. How then do the countries we have studied differ contextually and how are they similar?

The people and the economy

England has a population of around 49 million, with a high density. Scotland and Sweden, by contrast, have much lower populations – around five million and nine million respectively – and rather low population densities (Table 2.1). While both countries have large centres of population, for example in the central belt of Scotland between Glasgow and Edinburgh and in the large metropolitan areas of Stockholm, Göteborg and Malmö, they also have large areas of sparsely populated countryside, mainly in the north.

Like all countries in Europe, England, Scotland and Sweden are experiencing low and declining fertility rates. The Swedish rate has varied greatly in recent years. After several decades of decline – to 1.6 in 1983 – it increased in the 1980s. By 1990, Sweden had the highest fertility rate in the European Union (EU), just above the level needed for population replacement (2.13), to reach the highest level in Europe (Table 2.1). This led some commentators to conclude that strong support programmes for families with working parents were one way to boost fertility. But then the fertility rate fell: over the 1990s it declined by a quarter, to the lowest rate since records began in the 18th century and the same as the average for the EU. Explanations for this include the severe economic downturn in the early 1990s and cutbacks in the social support system (Gunnarsson et al, 1999).

The UK had a lower birth rate in 1990 (1.83). But over the decade the UK rate fell less than Sweden's, so that it finished slightly ahead of Sweden in 2000. While the overall populations of both Sweden and the UK are expected to rise slightly between 2000 and 2015, the child population (under-15s) is expected to fall in this period (Table 2.1).

Table 2.1: Population statistics in England, Scotland, UK and Sweden

	Population (millions) (2001)	Population density (persons per hectare) (1999)	Total fertility rate (2001)	Estimated fall in population under 15 years (2000-15)	Mean age of mother at birth (2001)
England	49.2	3.18	1.6	–	29.3
Scotland	5.1	0.65	1.5	–	29.2
UK	59.9	–	1.6	–11	29.2
Sweden	8.9	0.18	1.6	–18	–

Sources: Eurostat (2002); Office for National Statistics (2002); OECD (2003)

Within the UK, England and Scotland differ. The fertility rate in Scotland is lower, 91% of the rate in England in 2001. In addition, Scotland records a small annual loss of population due to migration compared with an annual gain from migration in England. Eventual population decline is not certain for England, with a projected population increase of 5% between 2001 and 2026 (Table 2.1). But in Scotland the population is already falling and is likely to continue to do so slowly, with a projected 4.5% fall up to 2026. Moreover the fall has been, and will continue to be, greatest among children and young people: between 2001 and 2026, the number of children is projected to fall 19% compared with a rise of 15% in people of pensionable age (Seenan, 2003). In particular, many of Scotland's rural communities face a steep drop in population. Fourteen out of the 15 rural local authorities in Scotland had natural negative rates of population change in 2000-01. It has been estimated that the gross out-migration of young people in these areas is around a third of the 16 to 21 age group (Bryden, 2003).

In post-industrial societies today, compared with recent history, women (and men) are having fewer children, later in life, with more women having no children at all. In England, for example, the proportion estimated to remain childless has doubled – from 10% to 20% – for women born in the early 1960s compared with those born in 1950 (Rendall and Smallwood, 2003). This is part of a complex process of change in the lives of individuals and in the structuring of family life, for most of which Sweden (along with other Nordic countries) has set the pace. Marriage rates have fallen and more marriages end in divorce; increasing numbers of couples cohabit rather than marry, with the proportion of those cohabiting highest among the 16-29 age group; more children are born outside marriage; and there are more lone parent families. On all but one of these counts, Sweden has the highest levels in the EU (or, in the case of marriage, the lowest level), though the UK rates are also rather high (or, in the case of marriage, low), well above the EU average, and the UK has the highest EU rate for lone-parent families (Table 2.2).

Sweden was until recently a very ethnically homogeneous country. But that has changed in the past 15 years with large influxes of migrants, especially asylum seekers: for example, between 1990 and 1995, 40,000 children between one and six years old were given asylum (OECD, 2001). By the turn of the century, a quarter of all children were themselves born, or had one or both parents born, outside Sweden. The largest group is Finnish, followed by large numbers born in, or to parents from, Yugoslavia, Turkey, Iraq and Iran. Moreover, 13% of children attending pre-schools in 2000 did not have Swedish as a mother tongue (Swedish Children's Ombudsman, 2001).

Exact comparison with the UK is difficult because of different methods of classification: in the UK, ethnicity is self-defined, while Swedish statistics are based on children's or parents' country of birth. But Sweden now has a large minority ethnic population, possibly higher than England, where 9% of the population defined themselves as non-white in the 2001 Census, with a further 4% Irish or 'other' white non-British. By contrast, and again in terms of the

Table 2.2: Marriage and cohabiting statistics in the UK and Sweden

	% of marriages in 1980 ended by 2000	% of couples aged 16-29 cohabiting (1998)	% of live births outside marriage (2000-01)	% of children living with one parent (1999-2000)
UK	42	53	40 (2001)	21.7 (1999)
Sweden	46	70	55 (2000)	17.8 (2000)

Sources: Eurostat (2002); ONS (2002)

Census, Scotland's minority ethnic population is much lower, with just 2% recorded as non-white. As in Sweden and England, the minority ethnic population is highly concentrated in certain urban areas: 6% of the population in Glasgow are from minority ethnic groups.

Sweden (with the other Nordic countries) has the highest level of female labour force participation among member states of the EU or, more broadly, member states of the OECD (including the US). Levels are high across the life course, with 78% of women with a pre-school child, that is, under six years old, in the labour force in 1998. The overall level for women in the UK is also relatively high, although lower than in Sweden, while the gap is greater among women with young children. Employment rates among this group of mothers, however, began to rise rapidly in the UK from the late 1980s (Brannen and Moss, 1998), some 15 to 20 years after a similar increase occurred in Sweden (Table 2.3).

One reason why 'childcare' services are more developed in Sweden than in either England or Scotland is the rapid expansion of it that took place in the 1970s and 1980s in response to the increase in employment occurring at that time among women with young children (Lenz Taguchi and Munkammer, 2003). Indeed, as early as the mid-1960s, 30 years before a 'national childcare strategy' was launched in both England and Scotland, "there was a broad consensus [in Sweden] among political parties behind the idea of building a national pre-school system" (Dahlberg, 1997, p 23). Service expansion was complemented by the introduction of paid parental leave for both mothers and fathers in the early 1970s (Haas and Hwang, 1999).

Table 2.3: Employment rates across the UK and Sweden

	Female economic activity rate (2001)	Part-time employment as % of all employment (women) (2002)	Employment among women with pre-school child (1998-2000)	Average hours/work of men employed full-time (2000)	Unemployment rate male/ female (2001)
UK	68%	40	53% (2002)	45.2	5.3%/4.2%
Sweden	76%	21	78% (1998)	40.2	5.5%/4.7%

Sources: Gunnarsson et al (1999); Duffield (2002); Eurostat (2002); OECD (2003)

An important difference between the UK and Sweden with respect to women's employment has been the position of lone mothers. In Sweden, both lone mothers and mothers living with partners have enjoyed high employment rates. By contrast, employment rates for lone mothers in the UK have been low, and they have also been substantially lower than for mothers living with partners (Bradshaw et al, 1996). This has, indeed, become a major concern for UK governments. The current UK government has set a target of 70% employment for lone mothers by 2010.

Although in most Swedish families with children both parents are employed full-time (Swedish Children's Ombudsman, 2001), many women work part time. The level is even higher in the UK, especially among women with young children (Table 2.3). Swedish mothers employed part time, however, generally work more hours than their part-time employed counterparts in England and Scotland: for example, most Swedish part-time workers with children under five years are employed for over 25 hours a week, most in England and Scotland for under 16 hours (Swedish Children's Ombudsman, 2001).

Around 90% of employed men in all three countries work full-time (and the figure is higher among men with children). But full-time employed fathers in the UK work on average 12% more hours than their Swedish counterparts. Indeed, UK men, including fathers, have the unenviable record of working the most hours in the EU.

As a result of recession, unemployment in both Sweden and the UK was high in the early 1990s, especially among men, for whom it was more than 10%. But after peaking in Sweden in 1997 and in the UK in 1993, it has fallen back in both countries and for both men and women to around 5%.

Employment in all countries is related to levels of education and qualification: the higher the level, the higher the employment rate. The gap is particularly large among women with children and largest of all for women with children under school age. In the UK in 2002, among women without dependent children, 88% with a higher qualification were employed, compared with 48% with no qualifications (a 40-point difference); among women with a child under five years the employment rates were respectively 72% and 23% (a 49-point difference). In 2000, among EU member states for which comparable information is available (unfortunately excluding Sweden), the UK had the second largest difference in employment rates between mothers with high and low levels of educational attainment (Escobeda et al, 2002).

This example raises two relevant points. First, the continuing rise in levels of educational attainment among women will drive up employment rates, especially during motherhood. Second, the large difference in employment rates between women with high and low levels of educational qualification is one of a number of indicators of high levels of economic and social inequality within the UK population. On most of these indicators, Sweden lies towards the other end of the spectrum, that is, social inequalities are much less marked. This becomes very apparent if we consider individual and household incomes, and it applies to the overall population as well as to children.

First, however, it is relevant to note that Sweden and the UK have rather similar levels of national wealth (once size of population is taken into account) (Eurostat, 2002). Both are relatively wealthy countries, with per capita gross domestic product (GDP) about 10% above the EU average, although only about two thirds of the US level. Yet Sweden and the UK produce very different levels of poverty from the same resources. The evidence is consistent and clear (Table 2.4).

Using a broad measure of poverty – the Human Poverty Index (HPI-2), made up of a number of indicators including income, unemployment and literacy – across the populations of 17 OECD member states demonstrates clear international differences. The UK has the third highest level of poverty, Sweden the lowest (United Nations Development Programme, 2003). The US has the highest level; despite being the wealthiest country in the world, the US is at or near the top on all international comparisons of poverty (for example, Luxembourg Income Study, 2000a; UNICEF, 2000). On a narrower measure – individuals with an income of less than 60% of the median, that is, the middle point in the distribution of income – in 1998 the UK had the second highest poverty level in the EU (21%), more than twice the level in Sweden (10%) (Eurostat, 2002).

The same picture applies to children. Data from the Luxembourg Income Study (2000a) show that the proportion of children living in poverty (here defined as 50% of median income) was more than three times higher in the UK than in Sweden – 15.4% in 1999 compared with 4.2% in 2000. The Swedish level was the lowest of 12 EU member states covered, while the UK was the second highest (after Italy). This wide difference between the UK and Sweden is confirmed by other cross-national comparisons (UNICEF, 2000; Eurostat, 2002). Within the UK, levels of child poverty are similar in England and Scotland (Bradshaw, 2002).

Looking in more detail at families most at risk of being in poverty, we can again see how levels of poverty are markedly lower in Sweden. In 1998, two-parent households with three or more children were more than twice as likely to be in poverty (defined as 60% of median income) in the UK as in Sweden (34% compared with 14%) (Eurostat, 2002). On a slightly more stringent measure (50%), the difference was similar for lone-mother families, with 34% of children in these families living in poverty in the UK in 1999 compared with 13% in Sweden in 2000 (Table 2.4; Luxembourg Income Study, 2000b).

These differences in child poverty are reflected in indicators of child health. The incidence of infant mortality, mortality for children under five years and low birth-weight babies, is twice as high in the UK as in Sweden (United Nations Development Programme, 2003).

The distribution of income over the whole population is also more equal in Sweden than the UK, whether judged against Gini coefficients or percentile ratios (Luxembourg Income Study, 2003c). In 1998, for example, the 20% of the population with the highest income in Sweden received an income that was 3.4 times higher that of than the poorest 20%, compared with 5.9 times

Table 2.4: Economic statistics in the UK and Sweden

	GDP per head in PPS[a] (2000)	Proportion of population living in low-income households (60% if median equivalised income) (1998)			
		Children below 16	Older people 65 and over	Two adults with three or more children	Single parent and child
UK	23,600	26	40	34	45
Sweden	23,000	11	7	14	19

Note: [a] Purchasing power standards, which enables a comparison to be made between countries taking account of varying price levels and exchange rates.

Sources: Eurostat (2002)

higher in the UK (Eurostat, 2002). The same is true of income inequality among children. In 1999, a third of children in the UK (31%) lived in households with extremes of income (either less than 50% of the median or more than 150%), twice as many as Sweden (15%) (Luxembourg Income Study, 2003d).

Overall, Sweden (along with other Nordic countries) has the most equal distribution of disposable income in the world, and this remains the case even after some growth in income inequality since 1997 (Fritzell, 1999; Kommittén Välfärdsbokslut, 2000; Abrahamson, 2002). Indeed, this growth of inequality has occurred only after the end of the economic recession, while "the recession itself passed by with surprisingly minor changes in income inequality" (Kommittén Välfärdsbokslut, 2000, p 108). This is not to say that in Sweden the recession left families with children unscathed. The proportion of children in families with a low income (below the threshold for receipt of social assistance) rose from 12% in 1993 to 21% in 1996, partly due to cuts in social welfare. However, the proportion fell again over the next two years, to reach 14% by 1998 (Swedish Children's Ombudsman, 2001).

Why does Sweden so outperform the UK? Esping-Andersen et al (2001) argue that mothers' employment is central to any policy approach to reducing child poverty. They conclude that "Nordic poverty rates are systematically low ... primarily because fathers and mothers are gainfully employed and adequately paid" (Esping-Andersen et al, 2001, p 65): the extensive provision of services providing childcare has played an important role in supporting high levels of parental employment. But there are other reasons why there is less poverty in Sweden than in the UK. The reference to adequate pay is important. Child poverty is higher where earnings inequalities are higher (Esping-Andersen et al, 2001). It is relevant therefore that the UK has the highest proportion of low-paid full-time workers in the EU, Sweden the lowest (Marx, 1999; UNICEF, 2000). Furthermore, Sweden, through its welfare regime (discussed below) has stronger redistributive policies, which also has a significant impact on the proportion of poor people:

> Before social benefits are taken into account, Ireland, Sweden and the United Kingdom show a high percentage (more than 30%) of people on low incomes.... Social benefits reduce the percentage of people at risk of poverty in all Member States but to very disparate degrees. The reduction is smallest – less than 30% – in Greece, Spain, Italy and Portugal. In other member states it is typically between 30-50%; in Denmark and Sweden the reduction is more than 70%.... It is notable that Denmark and Sweden have some of the lowest at-risk-of-poverty rates after payment of pensions and other benefits.... Ireland and the United Kingdom have some of the highest 'at risk of poverty' rates in the EU before benefits, and the inequalities remain higher than the Community average after payment of benefits (but the benefits have nevertheless had some redistributive effect). (Eurostat, 2002, p 92)

Differences in distributive policies have also affected the extent to which inequalities have increased over time. Esping-Andersen et al (2001) point out that demographic factors, such as the rise of more vulnerable households and changes in labour markets, including more precarious employment and increasing earnings disparities, are producing a long-term and structural trend towards an increase in market inequalities. Consequently in most countries, primary income inequality, that is, income *before* tax and benefits, has increased by between 10% and 30% – but this is not necessarily replicated in final disposable income, that is, income *after* tax and benefits. Thus, from the 1980s to the mid-1990s, primary income inequality actually increased more in Sweden than the UK (by 25% compared with 9%), but the situation was reversed for disposable income, for which inequality rose just 1% in Sweden compared with 14% in the UK: public redistribution over this period increased in Sweden but fell in the UK. Overall, Esping-Andersen et al (2001, p 26) conclude, "the Nordic countries are among the few OECD countries able to sustain *both* aged and child poverty at reasonably low levels".

The conclusion is clear. Sweden "secures minimal child poverty by its *combined strategy* of generous transfers and support for working mothers ... (while in the UK) families depend far more on either the male breadwinner or on transfers" (Esping-Andersen et al, 2001, p 73). Since 1997, the UK government has attached high priority to reducing child poverty; the Prime Minister has pledged to eradicate it by 2020 (though reducing income inequality does not figure as a target). To some extent, the UK government is adopting a Swedish approach, stimulating maternal employment through increasing 'childcare' services (although, unlike Sweden, as we shall see in Chapter Four, services are expected not only to enable mothers to work but to reduce poverty by breaking a presumed 'cycle of deprivation' through 'early intervention') and increasing cash transfers. There are no recent comparisons for Sweden and the UK of the redistributive effects of post-1997 transfer policies. But policies on services remain very different as between Sweden and the UK, despite the UK government's new-found concern to increase 'childcare' services. In a nutshell, to be expanded in Chapter Five, Sweden provides a universal entitlement to low-cost services, while the UK targets public support to lower-income parents using childcare, reaching a small proportion of the total population.

Whether the UK's anti-poverty strategy succeeds in the long term remains to be seen. Some progress has been made. There has been improvement in terms of ownership of certain items, problem debts and housing. The proportion of children in families suffering from hardship so measured fell between 1999 and 2001 from 47% to 33%, and from 28% to 15% for multiple hardship (Vegeris and Perry, 2003). The proportion of children living in low-income families has also fallen. After continuing to rise in the first two years of the Labour government, by 2001-02 the numbers of children in poverty had dropped by around half a million to the lowest level recorded since 1991 (Brewer et al, 2003). Out-of-work benefits to families with dependent children have risen by about 30% in real terms since 1998, but the main reason for falling poverty has been falling unemployment (Palmer et al, 2003).

It has been estimated that by 2004 child poverty will have dropped further and that "the Government's target (of reducing child poverty by a quarter by 2004-5) should be met" (Sutherland et al, 2003, p 3). Halving child poverty by 2010 "will require substantially more redistribution to the poorest ... (and) further reductions in child poverty are likely to be increasingly hard to achieve" (Brewer et al, 2003, p 5). Using a relative measure of poverty, that is, defining poverty in relation to average income, makes reducing poverty harder if overall incomes are growing, since this raises the poverty line.

Other problems remain. Unemployment has fallen, but not the amount of 'in-work poverty' arising from low pay (Palmer et al, 2003). This persistent problem is illustrated in a study of the impact of a local nursery in a disadvantaged inner-city area: more of the mothers using the nursery obtained jobs than a control group, but there was no corresponding increase in household income because most ended in low-paid employment (Evans, 2003b). Despite fewer people on very low pay, overall inequality in earnings continues to grow because of the fast-rising earnings of the highest-paid tenth (Palmer et al, 2003). In terms of income rather than earnings, the poorest tenth of the population has 2% of total national income, compared with 29% for the richest tenth. The Gini coefficient, a popular measure of income inequality, shows a considerable increase during the 1980s, stabilisation in the early 1990s, followed by a slight fall during the last Conservative government (1992-97) – but a further rise since 1997: "indeed despite the slight (statistically insignificant) fall in 2001-02, income inequality over the past two years has been higher than in any other period covered by our data" (Shephard, 2003, p 4). Reducing child poverty may, therefore, have gone hand in hand with increasing income inequality.

Welfare regimes

Esping-Andersen (1999, p 73) describes welfare regimes as "the ways in which welfare production is allocated between state, market and households". In recent years, increasing attention has been paid to classifying countries according to welfare regime. This has generated considerable academic dispute both about the criteria to be employed and the extent of differentiation between countries. Esping-Andersen's original work proposed a three-part typology of welfare regimes, which has been questioned on several grounds: "(as) a typology too narrowly based on income-maintenance programmes, too focused on only the state-market nexus, and too one-dimensionally built around the standard male production worker" (Esping-Andersen, 1999, p 73). A particularly strong critique came from feminist scholars, who argued that his typology paid too much attention to benefits and took little account of issues of care, which are of central importance to women.

Esping-Andersen termed the three regimes of his original typology conservative, liberal and social democratic. We will here focus on the last two, since the UK has a liberal (or Anglo-Saxon) regime, Sweden a social democratic (or Nordic) one. Liberal welfare states are characterised by targeted public policies focused on low-income groups and perceived 'market failures', that is, where market mechanisms do not produce the required result – for example, the population deemed in need of a service cannot afford fees at the market rate. Liberal regimes are also characterised by flat-rate, means-tested benefits, an increasing expectation that the majority will make their own welfare arrangements, and a strong move from public to private provision, promoting market solutions:

> There are three core elements that characterise the liberal regime. It is, firstly, *residual* in the sense that social guarantees are typically limited to 'bad risks'.... [It] is, secondly, residual in the sense that it adheres to a *narrow conception of what risks should be considered 'social'*.... The third characteristic of liberalism is its *encouragement of the market*.... [T]he residual approach cultivates dualisms: the good risks can be self-reliant in the market; the bad ones become 'welfare dependents'. (Esping-Andersen, 1999, pp 75-6; emphasis added)

While there has been no consensus in the literature about how many types of welfare model exist and where particular countries should be placed in the varying typologies, "it is fair to say that the 'Nordic model' has been the least contested of these groupings" (Kommittén Välfärdsbokslut, 2000, p 9). A Swedish commission of researchers, set up by the government in 1997 to review welfare developments in Sweden during the 1990s, emphasises that "an undisputed list of traits of what constitutes the [Nordic] model remains elusive" (Kommittén Välfärdsbokslut, 2000, p 9). Yet it is able to list a number of characteristics about which there is widespread agreement: the extensive scope of public policy, an emphasis on full employment and active labour market policies, a high degree of universalism, high benefit levels with an earnings-related component, relatively generous transfers and extensive services, and a high share of social expenditure in the gross national product (GNP). Esping-Andersen (1999) summarises the social democratic welfare state as committed to universalism and to:

> *comprehensive risk coverage, generous benefit levels and egalitarianism....* The social democratic regime is distinct also for its active and, in a sense, explicit effort to decommodify welfare, to minimize or altogether *abolish market dependency....* [What] is uniquely social democratic is, firstly, the fusion of universalism with generosity and, secondly, its comprehensive socialization of risks. (Esping-Andersen, 1999, pp 78-9; emphasis added)

Two other features of the Nordic welfare regime should be emphasised: redistribution and decentralisation "so that a significant part of the welfare arrangements are handled within the framework of municipal self-government" (Abrahamson, 2002, p 7). And whereas the market is the key institution for delivering welfare in liberal regimes, the state is the key institution in the Nordic regime (Abrahamson, 2002, p 7).

More recently, Esping-Andersen has attempted to respond to criticism that his initial study of welfare regimes paid insufficient attention to gender, family and care. He has widened his analysis from a focus on welfare cash benefits to include care services (for both children and older people). He has related the provision of services to the concept of 'defamilialisation', which "refers to the degree to which households' welfare and caring responsibilities are relaxed – either via welfare state provision, or via market provision" (Esping-Andersen, 1999, p 51). He sees the social democratic or Nordic welfare regimes as unique in their level of service provision, constituting "a distinct world of advanced defamilialization" (p 66; see also Moss and Cameron, 2002 for a review of service provision in Europe). At the opposite extreme are southern European countries, which have fewest services and 'appear unusually familialistic': familialism is a "composite of the male breadwinner bias of social protection and the centrality of the family as care-giver and ultimately responsible for its members' welfare" (p 83). Whereas conservative regimes tend towards viewing care as a family responsibility, liberal regimes "view servicing as a natural market activity, (and) as an individual responsibility" (p 76).

Esping-Andersen uses the UK as an example of how welfare regimes are not set in stone but can shift over time. He argues that an analysis in the 1970s would have put the UK and Sweden in the same grouping:

> [B]oth were built on universal, flat-rate benefit programmes, national health care, and a vocal political commitment to full employment. Moving ahead into the 1970s and beyond, the two clearly part ways: Britain failed to uphold its full employment commitment and to supplement modest flat-rate benefits with a guarantee of adequate income replacement. Failure to keep up

> promoted a gradual privatisation that was, no doubt, accelerated by concerted de-regulation, more targeting, and privatisation during the 1980s: sickness and maternity benefits were transferred to employers, council housing was sold off, the earnings-related pension (SERPS) was 'privatised' through opting out, and both private pensions and health insurance have been nurtured through tax subsidies. In a contemporary comparison then, Britain appears increasingly liberal. *Britain is an example of regime shifting or, perhaps, stalled 'social democratization'.* (p 87; emphasis added)

The UK's turn to a liberal welfare regime in the late 1970s was accompanied by shifts in economic and political regimes, again in a particular liberal direction. Economically, the 1970s have been described as marking the end of the dominance of a 'Fordist', or paternalistic, type of capitalism to be replaced, at least in the English-speaking world, by a capitalism variously characterised as 'flexible' (Harvey, 1989), 'free market' and 'disordered, anarchic' (Gray, 1998), 'short termist' (Sennett, 1998) and 'neo-liberal'. These new forms of capitalism attach high value to markets, competition, economic deregulation, flexibility, privatisation and commodification. Neo-liberalism and its attendant values have been most welcomed by the governments, and have had most impact in, English-speaking countries, in particular the US, New Zealand and the UK. It seems likely that this new economic regime played a major part in the growing poverty, inequality and social fragmentation that were so striking a feature of these countries in the 1980s.

This change in the economic regime was matched politically. Rose (1999) describes the emergence of an 'advanced liberal' state from the 1970s, linked to neo-liberalism in the economic field. The neo-liberal state is the successor to the 'social state', which had itself emerged as a reaction to, and a correction of, the failures of the 19th-century laissez-faire liberal state. A liberal orientation emphasises the distinction between public and private spheres, locating family and care within the private domain. It places value on individualism and independence: the ideal subject of an advanced liberal regime, as Rose points out, is the autonomous, self-governing citizen, active in making choices and willing to take personal responsibility for managing his or her own risks and those of her family. The role of the state is 'to enable a market to exist, and to provide what it needs to function' (Rose, 1999), which includes informed consumers, a degree of regulation and measures to tackle market failure. The possibility of market failure extends beyond the buying and selling of goods to the market for services, including education, health and welfare.

Differences in welfare regime are associated with differences in the way benefits and services are paid for and therefore how costs are distributed. Ask people in the UK what they associate with Sweden, and for most of them one of the first responses will be high taxes. This is certainly true. Tax receipts, as a proportion of GDP, are high in Sweden, well above the EU average (41%) or the UK level (Table 2.5).

But to say people pay more in taxes in Nordic welfare regimes is not the

Table 2.5: Tax and public expenditure in the UK and Sweden

	Total tax receipts as % of GDP (2000)	Public expenditure on social protection per head in PPS[a] (1999)	Public expenditure on social protection as % of GDP (1999)	Public expenditure on education as % of GDP (2000)
UK	37	5,872	26.9	4.9
Sweden	54	7,116	32.9	8.4

[a] Purchasing power standards, which enables a comparison to be made between countries taking account of varying price levels and exchange rates.

Sources: Eurostat (2002); OECD (2003)

same as saying that these regimes are more expensive. The total expense includes not only taxes paid but all other payments made for benefits and services, including private arrangements. Once these are taken into account, "expenditure on social purposes in the Nordic countries is no higher than those in countries with a Continental European welfare model such as Germany and the Netherlands, and does not even exceed the level of spending in countries with an Anglo-Saxon welfare model such as the United Kingdom and the United States" (Kvist, 2002, p 21). What distinguishes Sweden (and other Nordic countries), therefore, is not total social expenditure but the proportion of that expenditure organised by the state through both taxation and public expenditure on benefits and services.

Esping-Andersen (1999) has vividly illustrated how high taxes are only part of the story by comparing Sweden with the liberal regime of the US. Total welfare expenditure as a proportion of GDP is similar in Sweden and the US. What differs is the balance between public and private expenditure – what the state spends and what families spend. Swedes pay higher taxes, but Americans pay far more in private costs: for example, six times as much for childcare services.

A similarly large difference in what parents pay for 'childcare' services is apparent between England and Sweden. The average cost of a nursery place for a child under two years in England in 2003 was £512 a month (€732), and £476 (€680) for a child over two (Daycare Trust, 2003). Under the new system introduced by the Swedish government in 2002, the maximum sums a parent will pay for a nursery place are SEK1,140 per month (€123) for a first child, and SEK760 per month (€83) for a second child.

The difference between liberal regimes, such as the US and the UK, and Nordic regimes such as Sweden, lies, as Esping-Andersen (1999, p 176) concludes, in "who shoulders the burden, not the total weight of the burden itself". Moreover, the US system, with its heavy reliance on private fees and subsidised demand (that is, tax relief to parents rather than direct funding for services), seems to produce rather problematic services for children: much provision is poor, staff turnover is high and wages in care work are low. The

Swedish system, by contrast, delivers uniformly rather good provision, staffed by a well-qualified and relatively well-paid workforce. (For further comparison, see the documentation for the OECD reviews of ECEC in the US, UK and Sweden on www.oecd.org)

Generous public benefits and services certainly cost government a lot in Sweden. Overall, Sweden has the highest public expenditure on social protection (which includes healthcare, pensions and benefits to families) in the EU, whether measured as a proportion of GDP or as expenditure per head of population – – in both cases rather more than a fifth higher than in the UK. Total public expenditure on education is also high, well above the EU average and 70% above the UK average (Table 2.5). On the other hand, Swedes get a lot back from their high taxes. Swedish parents receive generous benefits such as 13 months' parental leave paid at 80% of earnings and up to 60 days of leave per year per child (up to the age of 12 years) available to care for sick children and at a comparable benefit level. They also have an entitlement to early childhood and school-age childcare services for children from 12 months of age – and, as we have seen, are charged low fees when using these services.

Furthermore, viewed broadly, the social democratic welfare regime has been highly successful, not least in areas such as poverty reduction, in which liberal regimes are still struggling, and as yet failing, to achieve significant results:

> Criticism of high taxation is placed into perspective when one takes the achievements into account. Judging the performance of the 'Nordic model', there is evidence of the success of the investments: low poverty rates, equal income distribution and progress in gender equality have been mentioned among most notable achievements. The Nordic countries score high in comparative indexes ... and fare well in international comparisons in the areas of education, social welfare and health. (Kommittén Välfärdsbokslut, 2000, p 10)

Once such benefits of high taxes are taken into account, and the private costs of alternative welfare regimes considered, it becomes less surprising that "the Nordic welfare states *enjoy broad public* support". Moreover, "it is the universal nature of policies that has arguably contributed to this" – and universal policies rely on high taxation (Kommittén Välfärdsbokslut, 2000, p 10; emphasis in original).

One other difference between welfare regimes should be noted. Over the years, the active involvement of the Swedish state in providing benefits and services has been matched by a willingness to regulate the labour market strongly in favour of parents and children. Parents now have extensive and flexible leave entitlements, backed by generous benefit payments. Sixteen months of parental leave may be taken full-time or in various part-time options down to one hour a day, and in either one bloc of time or several, at any time until a child's eighth birthday. Parents are also entitled to work reduced hours until children are eight years of age. Generous paid leave is available if children are ill. Flexibility is seen as working in the interest of parents, and its effect on the labour market is given a lower priority.

The contrast with the UK is striking. Here, successive governments have been resistant, or reluctant, to regulate for parental leave, which they have viewed as counter to the creation of a deregulated labour market. For neo-liberal governments, flexibility is defined in terms of employers', not parents', needs. When the state has intervened, it has been to introduce minimal standards. At the same time, the neo-liberal state (perhaps with a nostalgic longing for the paternalistic, 'Fordist' model of capitalism) has urged individual employers to supplement minimal standards with individual or company benefits. The upshot is weak entitlements for working parents. Since April 2003, statutory maternity leave has been extended to 52 weeks (far longer than anywhere else in the world), but for 46 weeks of this period leave is either unpaid or paid at a low flat-rate level. Parental leave is of short duration (three months per parent), unpaid, inflexibly available only on a full-time basis and only to be taken at the rate of four weeks per year. The most recent entitlement given to parents is the right to ask their employer if they can work reduced hours – not a right to reduced hours itself. (For a fuller discussion and comparison of leave policies in Sweden, the UK and other countries, see Deven and Moss, 2002.)

We have focused in this section on the two nation states – Sweden and the UK, looking at England and Scotland together. In some areas of welfare regime, such as social security and leave policies, this reflects the level where overall responsibility for policy resides. But in a number of other areas, such as health, services for children and families, and care services for older people, recent devolutionary reforms place responsibility with the constituent countries of the UK. We shall consider in later chapters how far Scotland and England are diverging with respect to children's services. But at this point we would observe that some decisions in Scotland, for example, over student fees and funding for personal care of older people, are more in keeping with the Nordic rather than with the liberal welfare regime.

Government

The historian Linda Colley observes that Britain evolved into "a markedly centralised state" (Colley, 2002, p 11), with a political system intended to produce strong government. The establishment of the Scottish Parliament, the Welsh Assembly and (in principle) the Northern Ireland Assembly has modified this picture. Yet, as we see below, strong centralising tendencies remain and indeed have in some degree been strengthened through the expanding role of HM Treasury in the policy areas and services that are the subject of this book. Moreover, if powers have been devolved nationally, local authorities have lost powers in England and Scotland to national government. This has particularly been the case in England.

With education in England, starting with the 1986 Education Act, the role of local authorities has diminished, squeezed between the devolution of powers to schools and stronger systems of centralised control – a national curriculum, national specification of methods – for example, the Literacy strategy – national targets, national assessments of pupils, and a new system of national regulation. A strong state has steered schools from a distance through increasing use of managerial techniques. The end result, as summed up by Whitty et al (1998), is an evaluative state and a quasi-market in schools. We shall see, too, in Chapter Three, how the expansion of early years education and care and school-age childcare has been guided and tightly controlled by central government, with local authorities given a limited role.

At the same time, there are signs of central government wanting to delegate more powers to lower levels of government and to institutions, prompted to some extent by a recognition that too much centralisation has proved counter-productive: we know, said a senior cabinet minister recently, that 'national targets work best when they are matched by a framework of devolution, accountability and participation' (Brown, 2003a, p 14). Some regional devolution has occurred in recent years, by means of non-elected regional development agencies with devolved budgets, in areas such as economic development, regeneration, skills training and business support. The government's 2002 White Paper on regional government in England offers the possibility of elected regional assemblies, if supported by local referendums, but their remit would not extend to education, care or health – crucially important welfare services. In order to let go of centralised powers, not only must government trust local authorities to act wisely, efficiently and in accordance with central government priorities; it must also be persuaded that decentralisation reflects key democratic values.

More freedom and less intrusive regulation are on offer to some local authorities and to some institutions, such as hospitals and schools. The same senior politician talks about opening up a "challenging agenda for modernisation and reform: more radical devolution of responsibilities from Whitehall ... with greater attention to the conditions favouring a new localism in delivery with greater transparency, proper audit and new incentives" (Brown, 2003a, p 13). He also argues that government's aim, in many of the new agencies and programmes – for example, Sure Start, which it has initiated – has been:

> ... a genuine break with the recent past: services, once centrally funded and organised, can and should now be led, organised and delivered by voluntary, charitable and community organisations.... This new direction moves us forward from the era of old Britain weakened by 'the man in Whitehall knows best' towards a new Britain strengthened by local centres awash with energy and dynamism. (Brown, 2003a, p 15)

This aspiration to a new localism is part of a tension at the heart of the current UK Labour government: between devolution and central direction, between equity and diversity, between decentralisation and control. Decentralisation is often highly conditional, a reward to be earned rather than a right. Detailed targets, inspections and other control systems remain in place. Detailed instructions still emanate from Whitehall.

The same tension can be seen in Scotland, which can still be subject to the views of 'the man in Whitehall' and has seen some similar trends in the centralisation of regulation and management of services. However, local authorities in Scotland have been less marginalised in the allocation of funding and subject to a less prescriptive regime than their English counterparts: we shall return to this subject.

In recent years, Sweden has gone much further down the road to decentralisation. It has left behind a tradition of centralised government that was reinforced by the almost unbroken rule, over 70 years, of one party: the Social Democrats. From the 1930s to the late 1970s, a centralised, rule-governed and bureaucratic welfare state was developed. However, from the late 1970s, a process of decentralisation began in Sweden (and other Nordic countries) that involved the devolution of responsibilities to local authorities. Unlike in England, therefore, in Sweden local authorities have gained in significance in the past 20 years.

Two examples illustrate this process. The first concerns pre-school and school-age childcare. Rapid expansion in the early years of the late 1960s and through the 1970s occurred under the centralised welfare state, and was marked by detailed state regulation of standards and funding. But in the 1980s, detailed regulations were done away with and more responsibility was given to local authorities. The state's role was reduced to providing more general guidance and support for development and research (Broberg and Hwang, 1991).

The same process occurred with schooling. In the early 1990s, when local authority influence over education was being reduced in England and, to a lesser extent, in Scotland, Swedish local authorities were given full responsibility for schools, including the employment of schoolteachers. This local responsibility, combined with responsibility for pre-schools and school-age childcare, facilitated the integration of schools and school-age childcare services, and closer relations between pre-schools and schools.

The devolution of powers to local authorities was paralleled by increased autonomy for individual institutions and more opportunities for parents to choose services. Rather than being a zero-sum game in which local authorities lost out to institutions and families, as in England, devolution enhanced the influence of all:

> As the municipalities became the employer of not only [free-time pedagogues and pre-school teachers] but also school teachers, their autonomy for decisions about these different groups of teachers increased. They became autonomous in setting financial priorities and determining the levels of teachers' salary. They could also make autonomous decisions on the management of teachers and pedagogical practices. Another change brought by decentralisation was that each school or pre-school was free to formulate and design its own pedagogical and methodological profile. In addition families in the early

> 1990s were able to choose between pre-school and school, rather than being assigned to the closest institution available. (Lenz Taguchi and Munkammer, 2003, p 21)

The national differences that exist today in the relationship between national government and local government are reflected in the sourcing of local government funding. The proportion of Swedish local government funding raised from local taxes is high in absolute and relative terms and has been rising in recent years: from 66% to 72% between 1990 and 1995 (Kommittén Välfärdsbokslut, 2000). A cross-national comparison in 1998 found that 80% of Swedish local government funding in 1998 came from local taxation. The proportion for the UK was just 29% – one of the lowest levels in Europe (OECD, 2002).

Three other differences in the context of government should be noted. First, Sweden has a long tradition of dividing government responsibility between mainly policy-making departments and national agencies responsible for the implementation of policy, including monitoring. Thus, the transfer of responsibility for pre-schools and free-time services from welfare to education involved both the Ministry for Education and the National Agency for Education (*Skolverket*). The National Agency website (www.skolverket.se/english) describes its main responsibility as "to work actively to ensure that national objectives for childcare and the school system are achieved". This involves it in a range of activities: collecting information, evaluation, supervisory and development work, and giving advice.

In recent years, some tasks have been delegated in England and Scotland from departments to agencies – for example, regulation and inspection. But there is still not the same clear-cut and well-established division of responsibilities found in Sweden, in particular between policy formulation and implementation. Combined with less local decentralisation, this places much greater demands on English and Scottish government departments. At the same time, however, these departments are marked by a regular and frequent turnover in senior staff who are generalist civil servants: there is a constant churn of staff, with little opportunity to develop an in-depth understanding of either the historical background of a policy or the issues that policy is meant to address.

Second, there are striking differences in the size of local authorities. England, with a population of nearly 50 million, has just 388 local authorities. Only 150 of these have responsibility for education and social services. Scotland, with a population of five million, has 32 local authorities, while Sweden with population of nine million has 289. Not only has power been decentralised to local authorities in Sweden, but these political units are substantially smaller, on average, than those in Scotland, which in turn are smaller than those in England. Thus, the smallest of the three local authorities in which we conducted our research in Sweden had a population of just 15,000. This authority was responsible for the same range of services as the largest local authority with which we worked in England, which had a population of 800,000. Yet, in the decentralised system operating in Sweden, the Swedish authority, small as it was, had more control over the children's services in its area than the English authority, acting as a direct provider of many services and the main funder of others.

Third, women play a substantially greater role in government in Sweden than in the UK. Women account for nearly half the national Members of Parliament (MPs) in Sweden, compared with around a fifth in the UK Parliament. The proportion of women in the Scottish Parliament – 41% – is considerably higher (and higher still in the devolved Welsh Assembly at 50%). At local level, 41% of Swedish councillors are women, compared with 26% in the UK (Eurostat, 2002). Given the different life experiences of women, including especially their relationship to care work and responsibilities, it is only to be expected that their different levels of representation in government might have some effect on policy for children's education and care across the three nations.

This higher level of political representation of women reflects the greater gender equality in Sweden than in the UK. Sweden ranks third in the world (behind Iceland and Norway) on both a 'gender empowerment measure' (covering political and economic participation and decision making, and power over economic resources) and a 'gender-related development index' (covering life expectancy, knowledge and standard of living). The UK comes, respectively, 17th and 11th (United Nations Development Programme, 2003).

Understandings

Increasing attention has been paid in recent decades to the theory of social construction, which proceeds from the premise that the world and our knowledge are socially constructed and that all of us, as human beings, are active participants in this process, engaged in meaning-making relationship with others (Dahlberg et al, 1999). For example, in the field of childhood studies – sometimes referred to as the 'new sociology of childhood' – it is now widely accepted that childhood is a social construction:

> Compared to biological immaturity, childhood is neither natural nor universal.... The immaturity of children is a biological fact, the way in which that immaturity is understood and made meaningful is a fact of culture. The facts of culture vary making childhood a social institution. Childhood is constructed and reconstructed for and by children. (Prout and James, 1997, p 7)

Meanwhile, Rinaldi (1999) puts the matter more simply: "childhood does not exist, we create it as a society, as a public subject. It is a social, political and historical construction".

Constructions – understandings – of children differ, and different understandings may apply at individual, group or national levels. While there may be diversity of understandings, particular understandings become dominant at particular times in fields like policy and research. These, in turn, affect more local understandings, but also shape provisions and practices. So our social constructions, our understandings of the child and childhood, are an important and productive part of context.

But they are also a particularly hard part of context to research. Government documents, for instance, rarely acknowledge, let alone articulate, such influences, presenting instead an objective veneer in which many things are simply assumed and taken for granted. This comment about the US might equally apply to other countries: "while much of the discussion [in the US] is about children, and in particular their poor structural position, there is no discussion about who children might be nor about childhood or the possibility of its social construction" (Moss et al, 1999, pp 25-6). Or, as Baker observes, in relation to the American (but it could also be the UK) public school, "much educational work flows around assumptions about children and their development – but what it means by being a 'child' is not debated" (Baker, 1998, p 118).

Thus, when we asked the informants in our study in England and Scotland whether they were aware of any discussions in policy documents about understandings of a number of key concepts, including the concepts of child and childhood, the general response was that such discussions did not appear in documents or, indeed, within government departments. One informant on secondment to an English government department, the Department for Education and Skills (DfES), said that meanings "are not debated or understood and there is no consensus about them. … [T]here is little shared understanding of key terms". This was put down to the pressure to get things done and "the government not [being] interested in meanings or debates". Another seconded official also referred to a climate in government that was not conducive to reflection. But he also argued the need to explain to officials why understandings might be important: "the debate about the child can be seen as a distraction … [It] is not helpful in short-term planning … [but] it is essential for long-term planning…. For a civil servant who has to write 20 pages for the spending review [an HM Treasury document] in the space of a fortnight, the debate is esoteric. You need to explain why it is important and why it should happen".

In Scotland, we found some discussion over the child and childhood among policy makers, centring on the notion that policy needs to shift from an embedded concept of children as vulnerable to a concept of children as more active and responsible. A Scottish interviewee noted:

> "Cultural attitudes … in the 21st century cannot keep taking demands and expectations of society and adding it on. We have to reverse the telescope and say the child is a resilient individual, the child is curious, the child is playful and becomes creative, is interdependent."

However, such comments were rare, particularly at a local level.

In such cases, it is necessary to rely, instead, on reading between the lines. We have to look for the concept of the child used by policy makers (or researchers or trainers or practitioners) by deconstructing what is said or written. In the absence of explicit discussion, it is necessary to search for implicit understandings. For this reason, it is this aspect of our discussion of context that is most speculative.

In the UK, both England and Scotland, diverse and in some ways contrasting understandings emerge. On the one hand, increasing reference is made to an autonomous and strong child, with rights, a voice and entitlement to participation. For example, Scottish education legislation now requires local authorities to 'pay due regard' to the views of children or young persons in decisions that significantly affect them and gives children the right to appeal their exclusion from school. Most recently, a Children's Commissioner has been appointed in Scotland.

A similar trend is evident in England. For example, the English Children and Young Person's Unit (CYPU) has now developed a set of 'core principles of participation' with supporting guidance (CYPU, 2001). These are to be applied across government, by all departments, and "provide a framework that government departments have agreed to work to in order to increase the effective involvement of children and young people in the design and provision of policies and services". Also, one of the stated principles of the English government's proposals for an overarching strategy for children and young people is empowerment: "children and young people should have opportunities to play an effective role in the design and delivery of policies and services".

On the other hand, a more problematic understanding of the child persists. The British media commonly represent children as victims or perpetrators, with an emphasis on bad things being done to children or children doing bad things (Moss and Petrie, 1998). Children emerge as dangerous and unruly, or as dependent and weak. This latter understanding, what Malaguzzi (1993) refers to as the image of the 'poor' child, is embodied in the language of the 'child in need' (a central concept in children's legislation) (Moss et al, 2000) and the 'child at risk' (the subject of a recent government Green Paper). Prout (2000, p 304) comments on this tension between different ideas of children, observing that "despite the recognition of children as persons in their own right, public policy and practice is marked by an intensification of control, regulation and surveillance around children". A respondent in our study, from the play sector, saw the same tensions when he described the growth of play space as a response to two contrasting influences: control (keeping children out of trouble and prevent 'hanging out') and enrichment (reflecting concerns that childhood has deteriorated in some ways).

Two other understandings of the child can be discerned in British policy, provision and practice, and appeared frequently in our interviews. One is the child as redemptive agent, the belief that powerful human technologies applied to children below a certain age (the current favourite is under three years) will cure a wide range of social and economic ills, in particular through saving the child from an adult future shaped by community disadvantage and inadequate parenting. Discourses of redemption and salvation "make the child an individual who is not reasonable, capable and competent but who – with the proper care and nurturing – can be saved" (Popkewitz, 1998, p 25).

This construction of the child is central to one of the most important recent UK government initiatives, Sure Start (see Chapters Three and Four). But it pervades a wider range of policy initiatives and interests a number of government departments. It also contributes to government's tendency to control, regulation and surveillance, since the belief in the benefits of early intervention, using proven technology, encourages a managerial approach that makes use of strong and detailed prescriptions of practice, standards, assessment and predetermined outcomes.

This technical, prescriptive approach is underpinned by child development theory, a very influential branch of scientific knowledge in the English-speaking world, in particular in early childhood policy and research. It provides a rationale for early intervention, a basis for technology – for example, developmentally appropriate practice – and a normative framework for monitoring and assessment. Respondents in England and Scotland frequently referred to 'child development' as a central concept in childcare and education. Behind the language of child development is a particular understanding or construction of the child, which has been termed the 'child as nature' or 'the scientific child', "an essential being of universal properties and inherent capabilities whose development is viewed as an innate process, biologically determined, following general laws" (Dahlberg et al, 1999, p 46). By implication, this child is an adult in waiting, representing potential human capital to be realised: he or she is that which is yet to be, a 'structured becoming' (Jenks, 1982). This process of becoming entails linear progress, as the child passes through successive, orderly and predicted 'developmental' or 'key' stages. The metaphor is climbing a ladder, or building an edifice on foundations. Each stage of childhood is preparation, or 'readying', for the next and more important stage, with early childhood devalued for its immaturity yet recognised as a necessary foundation for progression, culminating in the completeness that is attained in the state of independent adulthood. This child, therefore, is defined as lacking, deficient, passive, incomplete, underdeveloped – and the more she is so defined, the younger she is.

Differing understandings of the child have also been apparent in Sweden. Dahlberg and Lenz Taguchi (1994), in a paper prepared for a government commission, have argued that such differences of understanding have been responsible for the different practices found in pre-schools and schools:

> The view of the child which we call the *child as nature* is, for the most part, embodied in the pre-school, while the *child as producer of culture and knowledge* is, for the most part, embodied in the school.... [These different constructions have had] direct consequences on the content and working methods of

pedagogical activity, and in that way affected the view of the child's learning and knowledge-building. (emphasis added)

Such different understandings – or constructions – of the child, and the practices to which they gave rise, also produced tensions between the pre-school and the school:

> Over the 20th century the Swedish view of learning in pre-schooling became opposed to a traditional instrumental view associated with schooling activities, including teaching skills such as writing, reading and mathematics. The field of early childhood pedagogy, by embracing the pre-school 'golden age' of free play and development, set up a conflict between 'natural' development and discipline, or between emotional, social and intellectual learning and the teaching of instrumental skills and knowledge in schooling. Thus the integration of the two school forms in 1996 can be seen as the culmination of nearly a century of conflict between opposing ideologies concerning childhood, development, learning and children's education. (Lenz Taguchi and Munkammer, 2003, p 27)

More recently, another understanding of the child has emerged and become rather dominant in Sweden. It could be found in many of the accounts that we heard. This child is a citizen with rights and a voice that should be listened to. The UN Convention on the Rights of the Child is 'a burning issue' (Moss et al, 1999). He or she is an autonomous, self-determining, competent and active child. He or she is actively seeking to understand the world, and as such is a co-constructor of knowledge and identity. She is responsible for her own learning, a child whom, the curriculum stipulates, should with her teacher plan her school day and evaluate her own work and learning (Lenz Taguchi and Munkammer, 2003).

Lisbeth Flising (2002), in a report prepared as background for our research, discusses how Sweden can be said to be experiencing a paradigm shift concerning how we understand and create meaning in our lives. This change, she says, has great consequences for our view on children:

> Many teachers (but far from all of them) still represent the 'old' view of the child as 'the empty box' that is to be filled with content and the question-answer method is their most important pedagogical method. In this pattern the child is seen as helpless and without resources or potentials. Another way of viewing children that becomes more and more common is represented by for example the researcher Gunilla Dahlberg. Her basis is a social constructionist approach and she refers to among others Berger and Luckman (1966), Gergen and Gergen (1991) and Maturana (1991). 'In a social constructionist perspective phenomena in the world around (environment) are seen as socially constructed phenomena and man as an active and creative subject. This way of thinking contains the emancipatory potential which

means that we as human beings, as actors in our lives, can change ourselves through our actions and in the power of the result of our actions' (Dahlberg, 1997, p 21). (Flising, 2002)

This way of viewing the child:

> ... builds on the notion of the child as an active and creative actor, as a subject and citizen with potentials, rights and responsibility. A child worth listening to and have a dialogue with and who has the courage to think and act by himself. The idea that the child is an active actor, a constructor, in the construction of his own knowledge and his and his fellow beings' common culture is built on a respect for the child as a resourceful (resilient) and curious child – a child with his own inclination and power to learn, investigate and develop as a human being in an active relation to other people. It is a child who wants to take active part in the knowledge creating process, a child who in interaction with the world around is also active in the construction, in the creation of himself, his personality and his talents (Dahlberg, 1997, p 22). (Flising, 2002)

Flising points out that these ways of thinking about the child and pedagogy have been current in Sweden and in educational official documents since at least the early 1970s, though, as the quoted passage suggests, they are still not universally adopted.

What is less apparent in Sweden is the image of the 'poor' child, the child as victim, the child in need. The Swedish child is less likely to be poor materially or to be framed as 'poor' because defined as 'in need' by a system of targeted services. This understanding, however, does exist: poverty may be less widespread in Sweden than elsewhere in Europe, but concerns are expressed about the marginalisation of a growing minority and whether the Swedish (Nordic) welfare state is "able to integrate marginalised and excluded people; and to prevent processes of marginalisation and discrimination from arising and developing at all" (Abrahamson, 2002, p 12). But it plays second if not third fiddle to the stronger discourse of the competent and autonomous child, the child with rights and voice. It is striking, for example, that a report to UNESCO by two Swedish researchers on the integration of childcare and education (Lenz Taguchi and Munkammer, 2003) contains no reference to poverty, social exclusion, children in need or any of the language of the 'poor' child that would abound in any comparable report covering England or Scotland.

Social constructions are not confined to children and childhood. Institutions for children (such as nurseries and schools) can be understand in many different ways, as can the staff who work in them (Dahlberg et al, 1999; Moss and Petrie, 2002). Of particular importance to the subject of this book – new relationships between schools and childcare – are understandings of care and learning and the relationship between them. Here it is important to note a difference in understanding between the two British countries on the one hand and Sweden on the other.

Sweden (like many other continental European countries) understands this relationship within a context that includes the concept of pedagogy. Pedagogy is a theory and practice that can be applied in work with many different groups (children, young people, adults) and across many different settings. It starts with the whole child – the child with body, mind, emotions, creativity, history and social identity. But it is particularly relevant that pedagogy understands learning, care and upbringing as being totally inseparable: not separate fields that need to be joined up, but inherently interconnected parts of life (for a fuller discussion, see Moss and Petrie, 2002). Thus, the Swedish curriculum for pre-schools states that "the pre-school should provide children with good pedagogical activities, where care, nurturing and learning together form a coherent whole" (Swedish Ministry of Education and Science, 1998, p 8). Lenz Taguchi and Munkammer (2003, p 27), in their discussion of how most Swedish families now want early childhood education and care for their children from an early age, refer to parents expecting a "holistic pedagogy that includes health care, nurturing and education for their pre-schoolers".

By contrast, the context in England or Scotland does not contain this encompassing concept of pedagogy, which assumes the integration of care and education as normative. Instead, the public discourse constantly refers to separate concepts of 'education' and 'childcare', expressing a compartmentalised way of thinking that assumes the separateness of these concepts. However, a more inclusive school-based tradition does exist, which might be termed 'education in its broadest sense', to distinguish it from another tradition, 'education associated with the academic curriculum' (Petrie, 2002). The former tradition was recalled by this English informant, a researcher and former teacher:

> "We always used to talk that we did not need care because for us [it was] how we understood education – we didn't like 'educare' because for us education is care, education has always been about the development of human potential and that has to have 'care' and 'leading on'. You can't educate well without caring and a good carer can't care without offering some developmental potential. I've not come across a conceptual discussion of care in documents except education and care being inseparable. If you go back historically and look at education – back to Plato and Commenius – it embodies a lot of what people talk about as care. It's only recently that education has become narrowly interpreted about delivery of certain narrow goals. You learn in a social context and you can't address learning without looking at the social context which has more emphasis on the caring side."

But, as this respondent suggests, this tradition has been eclipsed in recent years by the other tradition, with its understanding of education narrowly focused on attainment.

Observations

We have reviewed some important contextual differences between England and Scotland (often, but not always, rather similar to each other) and Sweden (usually, but not always, different from the other two nations). This provides a framework for understanding and interpreting the accounts of reform that follow. It enables us to make some sense of similarities and differences.

We have shown that the three countries are following similar directions in terms of demographic and social change, although Sweden is often some years ahead of England and Scotland in terms of developments. This is especially true of maternal employment, which has had a place in, and contributed to, Sweden's developing policies from an earlier date, and of Sweden's more advanced provision of services (certainly with respect to early childhood and school-age childcare services) and leave entitlements. But there are other reasons for policy differences in these fields, in particular strikingly different welfare regimes that have produced very different attitudes to the respective responsibilities of state, market and family: the one emphasising public responsibility for universal provision, the other more inclined to limit public responsibility to targeted needs and the regulation of the private market. When early childhood and school-age childcare services were transferred from the welfare system to education in England, Scotland and Sweden, they brought with them, therefore, very different cultural baggage, which was in the Swedish case nearer to the culture of the education system with its principles of free access and universal provision.

The Swedish welfare regime also appears to have been quite successful in keeping levels of child poverty relatively low. While there are debates in Sweden today about social exclusion, these mainly focus on the rapidly expanding minority ethnic population. In stark contrast, because increasingly liberal welfare regimes in England and Scotland failed to avert a massive increase in child poverty and its associated ills, these two countries have relatively high levels of child poverty. The reduction of child poverty was high on the policy agenda of the new Labour administration when it came to power in 1997 after 18 years of Conservative government. This policy thrust had major implications for children's services and their reform.

Differences in welfare regime and the relationship between central and local government combine to produce a very different climates of governance in the three nations studied: private markets and a controlling state in England and, to a lesser extent, Scotland; public provision and local autonomy in Sweden. England and Scotland have a diversity of providers and types of provision, but the application of strong managerial systems by government ensures their conformity to various centrally determined norms. In contrast, Sweden has rather uniform services and providers, but considerable potential for the exercise of local autonomy, leading to diversity in organisation and practice.

The context of ideas or understandings also differs. England and Scotland seem marked by more variation and conflicting understandings of the child –

– between the poor child and the rich child, between the child as citizen and the child in need of control and surveillance. They lack a widely understood way of thinking that dissolves the borders between education and care; or perhaps we should say a way of thinking that does not create these borders in the first place. Sweden, by contrast, seems to have an increasingly clear and widely agreed understanding of what it means to be a child in a post-industrial society, and has access to an integrative concept – pedagogy – that encompasses education and care.

Part Two:
Bringing childcare services into education

THREE

England

Craig's story

Craig was born in 1996 and lives with his mother, Karen, in a council house in a city in the South West of England. The inner-city area where the family lives has a large minority ethnic community, and is also an area of multiple deprivation with levels of unemployment and economic inactivity higher than the average in England.

Craig's care and education from birth to seven years

Karen left school at 16 and worked full-time in a local café but gave up work to look after Craig. She was able to get financial support from the government, receiving a universal Child Benefit payment together with a means-tested Income Support payment that also allowed her to access Housing Benefit covering her council house rent and Council Tax. In total, her benefits provided her with 28% of the average income for households in England and Wales (before housing costs). When pregnant with Craig, she had been offered a government Social Fund loan to help with some of the costs associated with having a baby. As this loan would have to be repaid from her benefits, Karen declined the offer out of a fear of getting into debt.

Because she did not go out to work, Karen did not require outside childcare for Craig. But she did want to meet other parents and she wanted Craig to meet other young children. She decided to attend the local parent and toddlers group at the community centre for one session a week. There was a nominal fee of £2 a session (€2.86) to cover the costs of the room but, as the parents stayed with their children, they did not have to pay salaries for childcare staff.

Subsequently, Karen's GP suggested that she contact the local Sure Start centre that had just opened up. (Sure Start is a programme aimed at children under four years old and their families living in disadvantaged areas: it is discussed further in Chapter Four.) The Sure Start centre was able to offer Craig, who was now three years old, two sessions a week in its playgroup, and Karen also made use of the centre's parent groups to meet other mothers. These services were provided free of charge to Karen. About six months later, Craig got a place in the local primary school's nursery class, also free, for the remaining three mornings a week.

By the following year, at four years old, Craig moved into the reception class of the same primary school for the full school day (from 9am until 3pm). He had thus begun primary education six months before the age for starting compulsory schooling. Here the teaching was rather more structured than he had been used to in the nursery class, although the children in the reception class followed the same Foundation Stage Curriculum, recently introduced for children aged three to the end of their reception year. The Foundation Stage Curriculum covers six key areas: personal, social and emotional development; communication, language and literacy; mathematical development; knowledge and understanding of the world; physical development; and creative development. At the beginning of this reception year, the teacher conducted a statutory baseline assessment of Craig to monitor his performance in key curriculum areas of language, literacy, mathematics, and personal and social development.

Karen had begun to wonder about further training and perhaps going back to work, but was put off by the possibility of losing income from benefits. She discussed the options with the staff at the local Sure Start, who suggested that she contact a personal adviser on the New Deal for Lone Parents, a government employment scheme. This personal adviser talked through Karen's options and worked out how much better off she would be financially if she was in employment or pursuing training. Encouraged by this, Karen decided to do a one-year full-time vocational course in childcare and education, leading to a National Vocational Qualification (NVQ) Level II in Childcare and Education, which she hoped would help her to access employment in this field. NVQs are a way of accrediting experience in the workplace through demonstrating competence assessed against nationally agreed standards. There are five levels: Level I is for people with basic skills undertaking routine and predictable work activities; Level II – Karen's course – is for people working under supervision; Level III shows competence to work without supervision; Level IV is for senior managers and advanced practitioners; Level V is equivalent to a degree.

One of the key factors in Karen's decision to enter the training course was an offer of childcare for Craig. Her adviser was able to access £100 a week (€142.59) for her to cover childcare costs, and she was also entitled to an additional £15 per week (€21.45) training premium. This paid for Craig to attend a privately provided after-school scheme, from the end of the school day until 5.30pm each evening.

Craig's care and education today, at seven years old

At seven years old, Craig is now in his second year of compulsory schooling, but has been in school for three years. The school is close to his home and has around 400 pupils, making it one of the largest primary schools in the area. His school day starts at 9am, when his mother drops him off on her way to work. The school day is broken up by two playtime sessions which last for 20 minutes each, one in the morning and one in the afternoon, with 45 minutes for lunch at noon. Fruit and water are available for the children during the morning break, and lunch is provided for a fee (although many children bring packed lunches). Although many children qualify for free lunches in this school, Craig does not do so because his mother is in receipt of Working Families Tax Credit (WFTC).

Craig's class has 30 children. His teacher, Mrs Kay, is educated to degree level and qualified after four years' training with a Bachelor of Education in 1996. She earns £20,252 per annum (€28,960.36). She is supported in the classroom by two classroom assistants who are not qualified and earn approximately £5 per hour (€7.15), which gives them an annual salary of under £8,000 (€11,440). Though not qualified, one of the classroom assistants, Liz, who is 21 and recently graduated with a degree in sociology, hopes to pursue a career in teaching and wants classroom experience before applying for a postgraduate teaching degree. The other classroom assistant, Claire, is younger at 18 but is studying part-time towards a NVQ in Childcare and Education (Level II). Claire and Liz support the teacher by helping out with group activities, the classroom decoration, and the preparation of, and clearing up after, activities. Each year, Craig moves into a new class, with different staff.

Craig's primary school class follows the English National Curriculum, which is a statutory requirement for children aged from five to 11 and comes into force at the end of the Foundation Stage. It covers three core subjects (English, Maths and Science) and seven foundation subjects (design and technology, information and communication technology, history, geography, art and design, music and physical education). At the end of this year Craig will be tested by his class teacher in line with the national Key Stage 1 Standard Assessment Tests (SATs). Key Stage 1 covers Years 1 and 2 of compulsory schooling. The SATs are designed to help teachers assess pupils' strengths and weaknesses and to determine what pupils understand about a subject. Craig will be tested on his performance in reading, writing and mathematics. All schools then report their grades to enable central government to create 'league tables' of schools in England. From 2004 Craig's is one of the pilot schools in which the teacher will use the work he does throughout the year, as well as tests and tasks that the teacher herself chooses, to make an overall judgement about his progress. The intention is to help his teacher to plan Craig's learning to meet his needs, to stretch and develop him.

Karen, now with her NVQ in Childcare and Education (Level II), has managed to secure full-time employment in a local private day nursery. The nursery is one of three local private nurseries owned and run by the same woman (who had previously been a primary school teacher). The nursery offers all-day care for children from six weeks old and opens at 8am so that parents can drop their children off on their way to work. Most of the parents are dual-income professional couples who work full-time. The nursery charges £110 a week (€157.30) for full-day care for a child aged between three and five years. Karen has arranged to work from 9.15am to 5.15pm to allow her to drop Craig off at school on her way to work. She is paid £5.50 per hour (€7.87), which gives her a weekly salary of £168.03 (€240.28) (after tax). This is topped up by the government via the means-tested WFTC, worth £77.66 per week (€110.05) and the universal Child Benefit of £17.55 (€25.10), giving her a total weekly income of £263.24 (€376.43), or 54% of average earnings for England, and 61% of average earnings of the region.

Craig continues to attend the after-school scheme. Although situated in the primary school, the scheme is run entirely separately from the school and is also entirely dependent on parental fees. Karen pays £5 per session (€7.15). After school, at 3.15pm, Craig makes his way to the classrooms where the out-of-school club is based. There are around 50 children, who have the use of two classrooms, one for children who want to finish homework and one for play activities. Craig is given between 10 and 20 minutes of homework a day and he usually gets this over with before playing with his friends in the club, many of whom are from different classes in the school. He particularly likes being able to play computer games on the console brought in by one of the out-of-school club staff.

The club is staffed by five workers: a supervisor who is qualified to NVQ Level III in Playwork and four assistants, none of whom is trained. The supervisor earns £7 an hour (€10.01), and the assistants £5 an hour (€7.15). Only one of the assistants, Stewart, is male, but even this is rare, with men making up only 2% of childcare workers in England (and 14% of primary school teachers). In the evening Karen and Craig usually spend about 20 minutes reading in line with the government's guidelines. Karen also checks his homework and helps him with anything that he finds difficult – again, this is in accordance with government guidelines and is much encouraged by the school.

Craig's future care and education, from seven to 12 years

Craig will spend a further four years in the primary school until he moves up to the local secondary school when he is 11 years old. In Year 6, at the end of primary school, when Craig is 11 years old, his teacher will test him, using the SATs, on his progress in Key Stage 2. Stage 2 runs from Years 3-6 of compulsory schooling inclusive, continuing with the three core subjects and seven foundation subjects that made up Key Stage 1.

At the start of Year 7, newly transferred to the local secondary school, he will continue with Key Stage 3 learning goals, including the previous subjects but extended to include citizenship and foreign languages. He will again be tested at age 14, this time on Key Stage 3, his fourth national SATs since starting at primary school. Before the end of compulsory schooling, 16-year-olds also take GCSEs or similar qualifications. Most young people remain in education for at least another year, either in the same school or in a separate institution.

The background to reform: services and change prior to 1997

As we outlined in Chapter Two, the reform process in England inherited a very particular demographic, economic and political context. Its main features included: high levels of poverty in families with children; fast-growing employment, overall, among women with young children, but with some groups lagging, in particular women with low educational attainment and lone mothers; a liberal welfare regime, emphasising private responsibility, targeted state intervention and the role of markets; a centralised government and local authorities with large populations but limited powers; and an ambivalent view of children, with a public policy discourse that combines rights and participation on the one hand, with control and protection on the other.

A further aspect of the English context was a legacy of policy and services, which the reform process would either have to change or to accommodate. First and foremost, government responsibility for the services covered by this study had always been divided. Responsibility for 'childcare' (or, as referred to in the 1989 Children Act, the primary legislation, 'daycare services') for children of school age and below was with the Department of Health (DoH): this covered a variety of services including nurseries, childminders, playgroups, out-of-school childcare and holiday play schemes (see Glossary of terms). In addition to these services and the National Health Service, the DoH was responsible for a range of child welfare services including child protection, family support for 'children in need', 'looked after' children and a range of domiciliary, daycare and residential services for adults with disabilities.

We should say, first, that the main source of care that employed parents used for their children was, and continues to be, relations, in particular grandparents. This might be termed 'informal' rather than 'formal' provision, which implies a service not provided by relations but paid for, whether by family or state (Woodland et al, 2002). In England, parents with higher levels of education, working full time and in higher-status jobs are more likely to use formal provision; other parents are more likely to use informal provision (Mooney et al, 2001). These educational and occupational differences were also apparent in Sweden some years ago, but are much less apparent today (Lenz Taguchi and Munkammer, 2003).

In the field of formal services, daycare services were the responsibility of the DoH and provided mainly by the private sector. This private sector provision consisted of nurseries and childminding, which were mostly run as businesses, and playgroups and school-age childcare, mostly run as non-profit private organisations. Public provision mainly took the form of a small and decreasing number of day nurseries, primarily for children considered to have welfare needs, together with more therapeutically oriented family centres (most of which, however, were run by the private non-profit sector).

Playgroups had grown rapidly in the 1970s and 1980s in response to the limited availability of nursery schooling. The great majority provided a part-time service not intended to meet the needs of employed parents. But from the early 1990s onwards, places had begun to fall. The main formal service for employed parents in 1997 was provided by childminders, but with private nurseries fast overtaking them. The rapid increase in private nurseries from the late 1980s and through the 1990s coincided with surging employment among higher-qualified women with young children. Nearly all this expansion came from the private for-profit sector (see Table 3.1, p 73, for changes in levels of all forms of childcare and early education provision between 1989 and 2001 – but take careful note of the small print).

On the other side of the care/education divide, responsibility for early education had always rested with the English Education Department, alongside the much larger areas of compulsory and post-compulsory schooling and further and higher education. In 1997, the department was called the Department for Education and Employment (DfEE). Responsibility for employment had been added to the education remit in 1995, before which the Employment Department had been separate from the Department for Education. The DfEE was responsible for school-based education for children below compulsory school age, mainly in nursery and reception classes in primary schools. As we shall see, it had also inherited some childcare interests from the Employment Department.

By 1997, therefore, a system of services had evolved in England that was both diverse and fragmented. Some services were open all day, some part of the day; some took all ages up to five years of age, others took narrower age ranges; some focused on providing 'childcare for working parents', others on 'education', a few on family support; some were free, others relied entirely on parental fees; some were publicly provided, others privately provided, on either a profit or a non-profit basis. Some were the responsibility of the welfare system (the DoH and local social services departments); others were the responsibility of the education system (the DfEE, local education authorities and school boards of governors).

Up to 1997, the major role of public policy in childcare was to regulate private services. This role was reformed and somewhat extended – for example, to take in some school-age childcare – by the 1989 Children Act, which led to a new regulatory regime introduced in the early 1990s. The Act also confirmed a long-standing policy principle: that public provision or purchase of childcare services should be targeted at the relatively small number of children and their families who met certain welfare criteria. It consolidated these criteria into one broad criterion, placing a duty on local authorities to provide support services (including 'daycare') for 'children in need' and their families (for more on the consequences of the Children Act for childcare services and the use of these services for 'children in need', see Candappa, 1996; Statham et al, 2001).

The other side of this coin was that government considered the purchase and use of childcare services for other children, mainly those whose parents were employed, to be a parental responsibility, in keeping with a neo-liberal approach (see Chapter Two). While earlier post-war policy had been opposed to mothers of young children working (see 1945 Ministry of Health circular 221/45 or the 1968 DoH circular 37/68), by the 1990s the government had adopted a neutral stance between 'parental' employment and non-employment; it treated the matter as one of 'parental' choice, the use of the term 'parental' rendering the gender issues involved invisible (Moss, 2002). Parental employment was deemed a private matter, for parents themselves to manage with the help of any individual employers who judged providing childcare support to be in their interest: government's role was confined to *regulating* the private market in childcare. Adopting this stance of benign neglect, a minister in the Conservative government in 1990 commented that "our view is that it is for parents who go out to work to decide how best to care for their children. If they want or need help in this task they should make the necessary arrangements and meet the costs" (Cohen, 1990, p 35).

Another reason for government not intervening in favour of employed parents, already referred to in Chapter Two, was to maintain the level of labour market deregulation considered essential to a competitive economy in an increasingly neo-liberal global economy. Hence the consistent government opposition (from the early 1980s) to the adoption of a statutory right to parental leave, despite the extension of this entitlement in the meantime in almost every other European country (Moss and Deven, 1999).

Small policy initiatives in the mid-1990s showed the first signs of some policy rethinking. These were perhaps a response to the changes occurring in the labour market, in particular growing employment among women with younger children (which began to surge in the late 1980s), as well as mounting concern with high levels of non-employment and so-called benefit dependency among certain low-income groups, in particular lone mothers. These early initiatives, a dipping of government toes in the water, suggested no major impending changes to a model of parents purchasing private services within a childcare market. Rather, they extended government's relationship to the market: from regulating the market, they took government into improving its workings by attending to 'market failures' arising from the low incomes of some potential consumers and a supply of services that was in any case inadequate.

On the demand side, some financial support for childcare costs of low-income families – the 'childcare disregard' for families on Family Credit – was introduced in 1994. A supply-side scheme to support start-up costs of school-age childcare – the Out of School Childcare initiative – began in 1993. (Start-up or pump-priming funding offers short-term subsidy, the rationale being that some new services, especially those serving lower-income areas or families, require financial support until they are established, after which they are assumed to become self-supporting businesses able to operate unsupported in the market.)

The intention of both policies was to increase employment among lower-income families by increasing the availability and affordability of childcare. Significantly, they both originated, not in the DoH, which remained the custodian of the welfare role of childcare, seeking nothing to do with parental employment, but in the (then) Employment Department. Responsibility for these fledgling policies was transferred into the newly created DfEE in 1995. A very limited 'non-welfare' departmental responsibility for childcare had therefore arisen in DfEE before 1997, even though it was located in the 'employment' part of the new DfEE, separate from the 'education' part, which had had responsibility for pre-compulsory schooling in the public sector for many years.

Early years pre-school education had been a low priority for government during the post-war years. The commitment in the 1972 White Paper, issued by the then Education Secretary, Margaret Thatcher, to extend nursery education to all three- and four-year-olds whose parents wanted it (DES, 1972) was not met. Instead, provision in nursery classes increased gradually and unevenly across local authorities, depending on local political priorities. This was matched by an increase in four-year-olds admitted early to reception class (the first year of compulsory schooling).

But, as with childcare, new policies emerged in the 1990s, increasing public involvement in early education. The Conservative government announced a new push for universal nursery education in 1994. Significantly, funding was *not* to be confined, as in the past, to school-based provision, mostly in nursery classes. Now, it was to go to any providers – public or private – that could meet certain standards. The twin principles of policy were a mixed economy market and parental choice. The means to achieve policy was to be a system of demand subsidy, vouchers for parents who could redeem them with the service of their choice as long as that service was approved and available. Vouchers were introduced, on a trial basis, in four local authorities in 1996 (including in one of our study local authorities).

These measures can be seen as the culmination of a growing acceptance by government of the importance of early years education, that is, for three- and four-year-olds, stimulated by a growing body of research, reports and other advocacy. The promotion of early years education was accompanied by a growing official recognition of the potential educational role of childcare services. In addition to revamping regulation and redefining the welfare use of childcare services, the 1989 Children Act, via its accompanying Guidance, emphasised the link between childcare and education, at least for three- and four-year-olds. It included a section on 'Education in Day Care Settings', which stated that "the aim should be to offer 3 and 4 year olds in daycare settings experiences comparable in quality with those offered to children attending school" (DoH, 1991, para 6.40).

These pre-1997 policy initiatives in pre-compulsory education were, however, dwarfed by the policy changes under way in compulsory education. Starting with the 1986 Education Act, major reforms swept through the system: devolution of budgets and other responsibilities from local authorities to schools; the introduction of a national curriculum and national standards; regular assessments of pupils' attainment; the reform of inspection with the establishment of the Office for Standards in Education (Ofsted); more information on school performance for parents; open enrolment; the encouragement of new specialist types of secondary school, for example, City Technology Colleges; and increased access for poor children to private schools (the Assisted Places Scheme). These reforms furthered certain key policy values and objectives – parental choice, diversity of provision, school autonomy and improved standards in socially disadvantaged areas.

The key relationship that emerged from these changes was between central government and individual schools. Local education authorities were increasingly marginalised and diminished as more powers, duties and funding were delegated to schools, and central government exercised increasing control through new agencies and mechanisms. Whitty et al (1998, pp 20-1) describe the result of a decade of reforms as quasi markets – the 'big idea' in educational reform, seeking to make public services behave like the private sector – combined with an evaluative state:

> ... central government reduced [educational professionals'] autonomy and enhanced its own powers in a number of significant ways and thus strengthened its grip over the education services as a whole.... [Ofsted's programme of inspection constitutes] an astonishing degree of state surveillance of the English education system.

To summarise, key features of the field of study as it was in 1997 included:

- *Split departmental responsibility* between welfare (DoH), responsible for daycare/ childcare services, and education (DfEE), responsible for nursery and compulsory schooling. This departmental split was replicated by distinctions between childcare services on the one hand and schools on the other in nearly every respect, including funding, access, types of provision and the structuring and conditions of their respective workforces.
- *A fragmented body of services*, not only divided between the welfare and education systems, but with different types of services providing for different purposes and families. Day nurseries and childminders offered childcare for working parents and were mainly used by higher-income parents; playgroups and nursery schooling offered part-time provision for three- and four-year-olds, of little use by itself to employed parents but emphasising education and play for children; while a mix of other provisions, including family centres, was focused on providing a welfare service, mainly for poorer families.
- *Low levels of publicly funded childcare and early education*, in absolute terms and relative to many other European countries (European Commission Childcare

Network, 1996). Publicly funded childcare (apart from a small amount of demand subsidy via childcare disregard) was confined to provision for 'children in need', a small proportion of children. Levels of publicly funded early education were higher, but still modest in volume. Most early education provision was in schools. Nursery education took the form of one year's part-time provision of approximately 12.5 hours a week in term time only. A recent review of early education in 21 nations concludes that "the range of publicly funded provision was between 12.5 (England) and 48 hours per week, with a mean of 32 hours" (Bertram and Pascal, 2002, p 15). But much early education was (and is) accounted for by the admission of most children into reception class ('school proper') at four years old, despite a compulsory school age of five (itself low by international standards).

- *A growing marketisation* of all services. Childcare, always dominated by the private sector, became more so as growth in the 1990s was dominated by nurseries set up as businesses. At the same time, maintained schooling was increasingly atomised and treated as constituting a market in which individual schools were in competition with each other and in some cases – for example, early education – with the private sector. The government's role was to improve the workings of the market, enabling parents as consumers to have increased choice and make better decisions.
- *An increasing role for central government*, modest still in the case of childcare and early education, but substantial in compulsory schooling. It went well beyond the role of improving market functioning to controlling every aspect of education.

The background to reform: post-1997 policy developments

Childcare and early education

Departmental responsibility for childcare services was transferred to education in early 1998. But this was part of a larger process of change, one of a whole raft of reforms that followed the election of a Labour government, in May 1997, after 18 years of Conservative rule. However, as we shall see, there were also strong continuities in policy before and after 1997.

The change of government in 1997 had an immediate and very evident impact on policies concerning childcare, early education and schooling. For the first time in peacetime, childcare became a recognised policy priority, alongside education. It was seen as contributing to a number of high-profile domestic policy goals. These were the eradication of poverty (social inclusion), in particular through increasing employment; the promotion of gender equality; a competitive workforce and increased productivity (HM Treasury, 2000). Most recently, the government's interdepartmental review of childcare (Cabinet Office Strategy Unit, 2002) reiterates and extends the reasons why government now views childcare as a policy priority:

> The availability of good quality, affordable childcare is key to achieving some important government objectives. Childcare can improve *educational outcomes* for children. Childcare enables parents, particularly mothers, to go out to *work*, or increase their hours in work, thereby lifting their families out of *poverty*. It also plays a key role in extending choice for *women* by enhancing their ability to compete in the labour market on more equal terms.... Childcare can also play an important role in meeting other top level objectives, for example in improving *health*, boosting *productivity*, improving public services, closing the gender pay gap and reducing *crime*. The targets to achieve 70 per cent employment among lone parents by 2010 and to eradicate child poverty by 2020 are those that are most obviously related. Childcare is essential for those objectives to be met. (Cabinet Office Strategy Unit, 2002, p 5; emphasis added)

Childcare therefore appears almost as a cure for all economic and social ills; it concerns almost every area of domestic government. The policy aim, reiterated at the start of the passage just quoted, was set out in 1998 in the National Childcare Strategy: "to ensure quality, affordable childcare for children aged 0 to 14 years in every neighbourhood, including both formal childcare and support for informal arrangements" (DfEE, 1998, para 1.26). How has this aim been pursued?

Availability

Official statistics on childcare places are problematic. For many years, annual returns of places in registered services were made by local authorities. The last such returns published were for 2001. From 2002, responsibility for statistics was transferred to Ofsted, the new regulatory body but, because of difficulties caused by the transfer, no statistics were available for that year. When statistics were published for 2003, they were not directly comparable with those for previous years. In the meantime, the government has been receiving a new series of statistics from local authorities showing the number of new childcare places overall, and the net change taking into account closures as well as openings. This new series, although frequently cited by government, cannot be critically studied and evaluated by outside observers. In short, there is no reliable way of charting change from the early 1990s, or even 1997, through to the early 2000s, although we attempt some kind of assessment in the concluding section of this chapter.

Provision has undoubtedly grown since 1997. The government claims that, between 1997 and 2002, the number of children in childcare services increased by 547,000, and that it is "on track to achieve its Service Delivery Agreement to create 900,000 new childcare places in the private, public and voluntary sectors for 1.6 million children by March 2004" (Cabinet Office Strategy Unit, 2002, p 10). Most of this growth has not been achieved through public provision or *sustained* direct public funding of services. Rather, the government's aim has

Box 3.1: Meeting the childcare challenge

The National Childcare Strategy published in 1998 outlined the government's proposals for 'quality, affordable childcare for children aged 0 to 14 in every neighbourhood'. The strategy focused on improving three key areas:

Raising the quality of care: better integration of early education and childcare; a more consistent regulatory regime between education and childcare; new standards for early education and childcare; a new training and qualifications framework for childcare workers; more opportunities to train as childcare workers, including places through the New Deal (a UK government scheme to reduce unemployment).

Making childcare more affordable and available through the UK-wide Childcare Tax Credit for working families – part of the WFTC. It provided help with childcare costs of up to £70 per week (€100) for a family with one child and up to £105 per week (€150) for a family with two or more children (in 1998).

Making childcare more accessible by increasing places and improving information: diversity of childcare provision to meet parents' preferences, increasing the number of childcare places through National Lottery investment and education places through pre-school education grants.

been to stimulate the market to supply more private investment and places. The main role of government in "delivering new places [has been] through pump priming funds to encourage childcare business start ups, especially in disadvantaged areas" (Cabinet Office Strategy Unit, 2002, p 10).

A new means of stimulating provision has emerged recently, extending the use of schools: "the development of childcare in, or around, schools will help meet government objectives to increase childcare places and provide wider support for disadvantaged children" (Cabinet Office Strategy Unit, 2002, p 40). The government is anxious that this development is seen as part of a wider move – set out in its 2002 White Paper *Schools: Achieving success* – to develop an 'extended' schools approach: "this entails schools and their partners establishing a range of services and facilities on school premises for the benefit of pupils, their families and the wider community" (Cabinet Office Strategy Unit, 2002, p 42). This may involve the private sector – both for-profit and not-for-profit providers – in developing services on school sites. But the 2002 Education Act, which came into force in September 2002, also enabled schools themselves to provide a range of services, including childcare. Previously, although half of out-of-school clubs are situated in schools, schools had not been able to provide childcare services.

Extending the function of the school is 'a key feature in New Labour's drive to combat social exclusion' (Evans, 2003a, p 10). The government "want all schools to become extended schools – acting as the hub for services for children, families and other members of the community". Funding, however, will be concentrated on disadvantaged areas. The aim of this funding is to create a network of "full service extended schools, with at least one in every LEA [local education authority] by 2006". Each full-service school will offer a range of services, including "a core of childcare, study support, family and lifelong learning, health and social care, parenting support, sports and arts facilities, and access to Information Technology" (DfES, 2003a, p 29).

A second area of service expansion has been increased education provision for children under compulsory school age. An entitlement to part-time early education has already been implemented for four-year-olds, and an entitlement for three-year-olds will be in place by April 2004. In fact, by January 2003, 99% of three-year-olds were receiving early years education, with 88% in publicly funded places (ONS, 2003a). Like the previous Conservative policy, Labour recognised the private sector, as well as maintained schools, as providers of publicly funded early education, conditional on meeting certain criteria and standards: in 2003, 57% of three-year-olds and 23% of four-year-olds receiving publicly funded early education were in private sector services (ONS, 2003a, Tables 2 and 3). A market in publicly funded provision has been created, drawing in not only schools but also playgroups, nurseries and childminders.

A third area of service development has been the Sure Start programme. Begun in 1999 and heavily influenced by American research and policy – for example, the long-running Head Start programme targeted at children from poor families – Sure Start is focused on children under four years of age and their families living in designated disadvantaged areas. Run by local partnerships, local Sure Start programmes deliver a range of services including childcare, training for work and help with basic skills. Sure Start has a central place in the government's anti-poverty strategy; the idea is that it will reduce poverty by breaking an assumed cycle of deprivation through early intervention, supporting children's development, boosting maternal employment and strengthening families and communities. By the end of 2002, 522 programmes had been announced, with 300 already running: "the forecast is that Sure Start will reach 400,000 children by 2004" (Cabinet Office Strategy Unit, 2002, p 11). Lessons from Sure Start are intended to influence all children's services.

Affordability

The main means of addressing affordability of childcare has been the introduction of a system of tax credits (originally Childcare Tax Credit, replaced by the childcare element of the Working Tax Credit in 2003: referred to below as CCTC) to subsidise costs for low- to middle-income families. Rather than long-term direct funding of services, the government has therefore chosen to subsidise parents. The CCTC forms part of a wider system of tax credits intended to supplement the incomes of low-earning parents, and is a central plank of government policy to increase employment and reduce poverty.

Box 3.2: Sure Start programme

Developed from the HM Treasury-led, UK-wide Cross-Departmental Review of Provision for Young Children, the programme supports developing and running services for children under the age of three and their families, living in disadvantaged areas, on a basis which engages the local community. The programme's objectives are:

- to improve children's social and emotional development;
- to improve children's health;
- to improve children's ability to learn; and
- to strengthen families and communities.

However, a different funding strategy has been chosen for early years education, in which the voucher system (that is, direct subsidy to parents) initially introduced by the Conservative government in 1996 was quickly scrapped by the Labour government in favour of a grant paid direct to services.

These and other initiatives have led to substantially increased public spending in the area of childcare and early education. Between 2001-02 and 2003-04, the government has allocated £8.2 billion (€11.7 billion) to early education, childcare and Sure Start, which amounts to between £2.5 billion (€3.6 billion) and £2.9 billion (€4.1 billion) per year. Most of this (72% or £5.9 billion, €8.4 billion, over the three years) is to provide universal, though only part-time, education for three- and four-year-olds. The remainder is equally divided between Sure Start programmes (£1.1 billion, €1.6 billion) and direct spending on childcare (£1.2 billion, €1.7 billion): the latter is divided between a large number of funding initiatives and includes a large slice of National Lottery funding (about a third of direct spending on childcare) allocated through the New Opportunities Fund. Part of this childcare funding consists of a 'childcare grant' paid to Early Years Development and Childcare Partnerships (EYDCPs, discussed later), which covers the costs of these partnerships, but also some funding for Children's Information Services, training and 'pump-priming' (Cabinet Office Strategy Unit, 2002).

In addition to the £8.2 billion (€11.7 billion) to be spent directly on services in the three-year period up to 2004, a further £725 million (€1,037 million) will be spent on childcare through the CCTC. Introduced in 1999, by October 2003 CCTC was being claimed by 285,000 lower-income families in the UK (Inland Revenue, 2003b). This represents a substantial increase, of 62%, since August 2002, following the replacement of the Working Families Tax Credit by the Working Tax Credit in April 2003.

Even after this increase in take-up, CCTC will still affect only a small proportion of families, especially as it covers children up to 14 years of age and in a range of provisions including nurseries, childminders and out-of-school clubs. In the second survey of parents' demand for childcare, conducted for the

Department for Employment and Skills (DfES) in 2001, only 3% of all parents received CCTC (Woodland et al, 2002), a figure comparable to estimates made by the Inland Revenue (2003a), which administers the system: the recent rise in take-up would bring this up to nearer 5%. Most recipients (66% of the total in July 2003) are lone parents; in 2001, 10% of lone parents received CCTC compared with 1% of two-parent families. Moreover, the average payment – just over £50 (€71.50) a week per family in October 2003 – was low, under half of the average price per child quoted by Daycare Trust (2003) for nurseries (£128, €183, a week for a child under two years; £119, €170.17, for an older child) or childminders (£118, €167.31, a week for a child under two years).

Total public spending per year on childcare, early education and Sure Start averages out at around £3 billion (€4.29 billion), or about 0.3% of GDP. Less than a quarter of this sum (including tax relief) has gone into general childcare services. Viewed from another perspective, it has been estimated that parental fees contributed 83% of funding for day nurseries in the UK in 2002, and only 7% of these fees were covered by CCTC. Including CCTC and the nursery grants paid to nurseries for the education of three- and four-year-olds, public funding accounted for 14% of nursery funding (Laing and Buisson, 2003). Overall, therefore, public funding, despite some increase, remains low, with parents by far the main funders of childcare services.

Other policy areas

We have outlined the government's commitment to available and affordable childcare and early education, and the means it has adopted. Its approach to quality – including regulation, curriculum and staffing – will be considered later in our discussion of the integration process. But in considering the policy context for the move to greater integration between childcare and education, three other policy areas should be mentioned.

The first policy area concerns the relationship between *parental employment* and *the care of children*. The new prominence given to childcare in public policy has been motivated not only by policy aims such as reducing poverty and improving educational standards, but also by employment-related aims, including increasing employment – for example, the target of 70% employment among lone parents by 2010 – and supporting employed parents by enabling them to achieve a better 'work–life balance'. For the first time, at least since the Second World War, the government has abandoned opposition or neutrality in favour of unambiguous support for maternal employment: "the Government welcomes women's greater involvement and equality in the workplace and wants to ensure that all those women who wish to can take up these opportunities" (DfEE, 1998, para 1.6).

Under the heading 'work–life balance', government has sought to improve the support available to employed parents. Much of this has taken the form of encouraging individual employers to introduce measures for their own workforces; for example, from 2005 employers can pay employees a childcare payment of up to £50 a week free of tax and national insurance. But it has also involved extending statutory rights to leave for employed parents: a statutory entitlement to unpaid parental leave (1999) and paid paternity leave (2003) has been introduced; maternity leave has been extended (2003); and parents with a child under six years old now have the right to request a more flexible working pattern from their employer, including part-time work (2003).

The second policy area could also be said to break new ground. Since 2000, the government has been developing an *overarching strategy for children and young people*, supported by a cross-departmental CYPU and a cabinet Children's Committee chaired by the Chancellor of the Exchequer. The aim is for all government departments to work towards shared 'key outcomes' and to apply 10 common principles, namely, that all policies and services for children and young people should be centred on the needs of young people, be of high quality, family-orientated, equitable and non-discriminatory, inclusive, empowering, results-orientated, evidence-based, coherent in design and delivery, supportive and respectful, and community-enhancing. This strategy forms "a framework within which future policy making should take place. The framework is intended to cover all aspects of children's and young people's lives, so will be relevant to developments in the field of childcare" (Cabinet Office Strategy Unit, 2002, p 12).

If the first two policy areas reveal new directions, the third policy area, *compulsory schooling*, has shown more signs of continuity, although the recent initiative on the extended role of the schools is a new departure. Otherwise, policies introduced under the previous Conservative administration have been intensified, with increased emphasis on specialist schools, parental choice and competition between schools through quasi-markets. There has been a renewed drive on standards, linked to departmental targets, focusing initially on primary schools but now turning to secondary schools. In addition to setting goals, central government has prescribed methods, with the Numeracy and Literacy strategies that include literacy and numeracy hours each day for all primary school children, having a major impact on the work of primary schools.

The changing role of HM Treasury

This discussion of the background to departmental integration would not be complete without noting the changing role of HM Treasury, which has become an important actor in the childcare field. This reflects a major transformation of HM Treasury's position in government, from the limited although important role of directing economic policy to assuming broad responsibility for shaping, delivering and monitoring social policy across the field. This has involved the deployment of a range of new tools, in particular Comprehensive Spending Reviews, but also public service agreements, which define departmental targets, and cross-cutting reviews, which are chaired by Treasury officials and bring together all other departments involved in the subject under review. Started in

1997, these have included a review on children under eight years old, which led to the Sure Start programme.

HM Treasury regards childcare as central to many of its aims. It has become convinced that early intervention with children and families is an important part of its strategy to reduce poverty: the Sure Start programme was very much HM Treasury's creature. Childcare is also seen as an essential condition for increasing employment, which in turn is seen as an essential means in the achievement of a number of important policy ends.

HM Treasury's approach to childcare and early years education is shaped by a number of principles: parental choice; markets as, usually, the best way to deliver services (for a discussion by the Chancellor on when the public interest is "best advanced by more or less reliance on markets or through substituting a degree of public control or ownership for the market", see Brown, 2003a, p 2); public intervention in childcare to be focused on regulating the market and cases of market failure. HM Treasury is primarily interested in increasing the supply of childcare places – it has a target in its own Service Delivery Agreement to increase childcare places – but appears to be less persuaded by arguments about quality (an example of how departmental positions still operate even within a government priority for cross-departmental cooperation). One senior official (not from HM Treasury) interviewed for the study noted that different departments had divergent approaches, with HM Treasury's interest in the volume of childcare leading to an unwillingness to engage in discussions about quality and a willingness to settle for 'good enough' provision.

Within the Labour government, HM Treasury has adopted a proactive role to stimulate childcare provision. It plays a direct role (across the UK) through responsibility for the CCTC, which forms an important part of the government's childcare strategy. This means of injecting public money into the childcare sector was chosen by the Chancellor for its compatibility with HM Treasury's favoured market approach and because it fitted into the tax credit system constructed by the Chancellor to reduce poverty and 'make work pay'.

But HM Treasury's role is broader. In particular through the 2002 Comprehensive Spending Review, it has set the policy framework for the development of general childcare services, as well as for more integrated services in disadvantaged areas (Children's Centres, to be discussed later). In his 2003 Budget Statement, the Chancellor reasserted his continuing leadership in this field when he announced a further childcare review (following the one led by the Cabinet Office in 2002) as part of the next Comprehensive Spending Review scheduled to begin at the end of 2003. This review will focus on the quantity of provision, looking at how fast the sector can expand and what more needs to be done in areas such as childcare for school-age children and the role of extended schools. The significance of this HM Treasury oversight and direction of policy, with its particular interest in 'childcare', for the reform process will become apparent later in this chapter.

The reform process

The responsibility of the DoH for 'daycare services' was transferred to education early in the first term of the new Labour government. The decision to move responsibility was taken in 1997. Initially, an official from DoH was seconded to DfEE, working on the regulatory issues, especially the preparation of a consultative document on regulation. A Childcare Unit was established in the (then) DfEE in 1998. Given the DoH's limited and mainly regulatory role in childcare, the transfer was not a major undertaking: the DoH ceded what was, in practice, a minor part of its territory. Because existing legislation did not specify a particular secretary of state, no legislative changes were needed.

Why did the transfer take place and at this time? Several factors were involved:

- *The cumulative effect of many years' advocacy.* A large number of reports over many years advocated the need for an integrated, education-based early years service, on the basis that care and education for young children are inseparable.
- *Twenty years or more of developments on the ground.* There were a number of local initiatives on integration, involving both individual services (for example, Combined Centres going back to the 1970s) and local authorities integrating responsibility within education departments from the late 1980s (for example, Manchester, Islington, Camden).
- *The increasing overlap between childcare and schools in early education.* During the 1990s, policy moved to the view that early education could be delivered in childcare settings as well as in schools. As we have already described, this was a necessary condition for the development of a 'mixed economy' approach to early education, foregrounding parental choice and a market approach.
- *Pre-1997 policy changes.* By 1997, DfEE already had some policy responsibility for childcare through the Conservative government childcare policy initiatives of the mid-1990s. It was also significant that, by 1997, it was the Department for Education *and* Employment. With childcare part of an employment agenda, there was a strong rationale for putting it in DfEE, although not necessarily integrated with education.
- *The commitment and influence of a key politician.* Margaret Hodge (with a background as a council leader in a local authority that had a history of integration) was given the task by the then shadow education secretary of developing the Labour Party's early years policy prior to the election, which she did with the help of a working group. A detailed policy statement published shortly before the election proposed an 'integrated and coherent early years service' (Labour Party, 1997). Hodge personally believed that 'education should be at the heart' of this service. After the election, although not immediately made a minister, she remained active in pressing the case for childcare being in education.
- *No significant opposition to transfer.* Childcare was not a DoH priority, and limited resources were devoted to its mainly regulatory role; for example,

there was just one person in the SSI for early years, devoting one day a week to the subject. The DoH had never been involved in stimulating, delivering or funding general childcare services. The DoH therefore did not resist the transfer, and indeed saw it as a positive move. More generally, there was no significant opposition outside government to the transfer, either from other political parties or from other organisations representing particular interests.

The transfer was, therefore, driven or at least facilitated by the conjunction of a variety of favourable conditions: the existing structure of government (with employment and education in the same department); the arguments for, and increasing practice of, close relationships between childcare and education (locally and nationally); an absence of departmental and other opposition; the incoming government's policy commitment in opposition; and a committed and effective politician who believed in the case. However, some of these conditions favouring integration proved transitory: the influential politician, after an energetic period steering early years and childcare reform, was promoted to another post; and the DfEE became the DfES, losing employment to another department, the Department for Work and Pensions (DWP).

Moreover, HM Treasury's interest in childcare as a means to further employment and reduce poverty, which has been a powerful driver of policy, does not extend to the view that childcare and education have a special relationship. It is concerned primarily with finding the most effective ways to create more 'childcare' places. A Treasury official interviewed for the study noted that HM Treasury sees childcare as a cross-departmental issue, with other departments having an interest wherever administrative responsibility is located. This view is reiterated in the recent interdepartmental childcare review (published by DfES, DWP, HM Treasury, the Women and Equality Unit and the Cabinet Office Strategy Unit), which notes that "at the centre there are a number of Government Departments that have an interest in childcare policy: DfES, Department of Work and Pensions, Department of Trade and Industry, Inland Revenue, Department for Culture, Media and Sport, Department of Health, Home Office, Women and Equality Unit, Office of the Deputy Prime Minister" (Cabinet Office Strategy Unit, 2002, p 49).

The issue that arises is the significance of the location of responsibility for a particular policy field, in this case childcare. Is location simply a pragmatic choice to be made between several potential departments, each with an interest in childcare, and of no more than bureaucratic interest? Or does location involve a choice of principle based on a clear idea of the policy field, which implies a special and privileged relationship between the policy field and a particular department? It could be said, for instance, that a number of departments have an interest in schooling; but there is no question that its proper home is within education. This is an issue we will return to in more detail in our concluding chapter.

The extent of integration at the national level

Departmental responsibility

The starting point for the study was the integration of departmental responsibility for childcare and education within the education system. In this section we consider how much further the integration between childcare and education has gone since 1997. But first we want to dwell on the issue of departmental integration, to see what in practice this has entailed. For, as we have just suggested, the issue of departmental integration may be more than simply a bureaucratic exercise. The location of responsibility in government and the way that responsibility is exercised may also be of strong symbolic significance, telling us how government and policy makers think about a policy field and its relationship to others.

The post-1997 history of departmental integration is marked by restlessness. An informant involved in the transfer of responsibility recalled there were some initial debates about boundaries – 'meat and drink to civil servants' – including whether to put childcare for younger and older children together (which they were) and what should be the upper end for childcare (14 years old was eventually agreed). The initial administrative integration was tentative and incomplete: childcare and early education might be within one department, but responsibility remained split between a Childcare Unit and an Early Years Division that dealt with education for three- and four-year-olds. Childcare was in the employment part of DfEE, early years education in schools, leading to cultural, organisational and budgetary differences. In addition, a new cross-departmental body – the Sure Start Unit – was also located in DfEE (although separate from childcare and early education) to run the new Sure Start programme.

Subsequently, after an internal review, it was agreed to merge the childcare and early education parts into an Early Years and Childcare Unit – but as a '*joint* unit' with two heads, rather than as a 'single unit' (each head took responsibility for different issues, for example, increasing places and matters to do with quality). The unit originally reported up through both the employment and schools sides of the DfEE. But when employment was removed to another department (DWP), the unit reported through schools. Following the second Comprehensive Spending Review in 2002, further changes occurred. In December 2002, the joint unit merged with the Sure Start programme. The resulting new unit was called the Sure Start Unit. There was at last a *single* unit with one head.

This unit, however, is no longer solely the responsibility of the DfES. For, at the moment when administrative integration was fully achieved, political responsibility was split. The Sure Start Unit was established as an inter-departmental unit reporting to two departments: education, as before, but now also employment in the form of the DWP. The minister responsible for the unit is described as 'the Minister for Sure Start in DfES and DWP'. The rationale is 'to ensure our early years and childcare vision delivers on both our educational and employment objectives', as well as to reduce confusion to parents and providers arising from 'differently named and separately branded initiatives' (Cabinet Office Strategy Unit, 2002, p 13).

The result of a five-year process of departmental reorganisation is that childcare and early years are now firmly located within one administrative structure, along with the Sure Start programme targeted at disadvantaged children and families. The structure has assumed the name of one of its constituent parts – Sure Start – a programme targeted at poor families. At the same time, the whole range of childcare and early years services has become, again, the responsibility of two departments – with employment replacing welfare as the partner of education. The structure may be different from before – a single administrative unit, with interdepartmental control and one responsible minister – but responsibility is nevertheless again divided between departments with different agendas and perspectives.

This most recent reorganisation is the latest twist in a long-standing debate about where 'childcare' should go and how it should relate to education. Indeed, several respondents in our study observed that after the 2001 election childcare might well have been located entirely within the DWP, reflecting the view of some (one informant referred to this as 'HM Treasury option') that childcare was primarily concerned with employment (rather than education). A civil servant recalled that "there was discussion that DWP would take over childcare because government attaches great importance to [childcare's contribution to] the labour market role and poverty agenda.... [T]here was some risk that work in stitching the Unit together might be pulled apart again". While the 'struggle to remain within education' was successful, the way was prepared for future cross-departmental responsibility. A formal relationship on childcare was established between DfES and DWP, with an agreement on joint working arrangements (including an Early Years and Childcare Joint Board with membership from both departments) and protocols.

Other areas of integration

Funding

Integration has gone furthest in provision for three- to five-year-olds, driven by a concern to develop a mixed economy and quasi-market in the early education field and to provide increased continuity between early education (for three- and four-year-olds) and the first year of compulsory schooling (for five-year-olds). The 'nursery education grant' provides funding across all services (including schools, playgroups, nurseries and childminding) providing early education. To be eligible for grants, they must meet certain conditions, in particular to be registered with Ofsted and to agree to work towards the early learning goals (both discussed later). However, the grant is limited to part-time provision for three- and four-year-olds in term time, amounting to 12 hours a week over three 11-week terms, that is, 412 hours a year. (See Box 3.3 for more about how the nursery education grant worked in the local authority where this day nursery was located.)

Apart from this limited entitlement, funding remains divided; indeed, it has become more so with the expansion of demand subsidy through the tax credit system. Schooling is free but childcare is paid for by parents, except for: (a) the small number of children provided with services because they are deemed 'in need' under the terms of the 1989 Children Act; and (b) the rather larger number of children whose parents receive some fee subsidy for childcare through CCTC, the childcare element of the WFTC. As already noted, the main form of public funding (excluding nursery education grant and the Sure Start programme) comes through this demand subsidy route. But in addition there is a plethora of funding streams (over 40 in 2002, according to the Daycare Trust) to support various aspects of early education and childcare development. Finally, the role of the National Lottery, in particular the New Opportunities Fund (NOF), should be noted, adding yet another funder and funding stream. NOF has been used UK-wide to stimulate a number of services (for example, school-age childcare, study support, and play opportunities), but on a short-term, pump-priming basis. Perhaps unsurprisingly, this plethora of funding mechanisms led the government's recent childcare review to conclude that "current funding and delivery mechanisms are too complex ... [with] too many uncoordinated programmes relating to childcare which have their own funding streams" (Cabinet Office Strategy Unit, 2002, p 13).

Curriculum

Developed by the Qualifications and Curriculum Authority (QCA) and introduced in September 2000, the Foundation Stage (FS) is "a recognised stage of education relating to children from 3 years old to the end of reception year in primary school", that is, over a three-year period including the first year of compulsory schooling and the two preceding years (QCA, 2000). All providers receiving a nursery education grant must agree to work towards the early learning goals (which replace the desirable learning outcomes introduced by the Conservative government) as set out in the Curriculum guidance for the FS. The FS therefore covers both childcare and school-based provision: it is, however, concerned only with a narrow age range of young children, covering a three-year period.

With regard to guidance as to what and how children should learn, the situation differs for children younger and older than the FS age group. At the end of 2002, a framework of effective practice to support staff working with children aged under three years was published (Sure Start Unit, 2003a). Initiated and funded by DfES, the framework has been distributed to 300,000 settings, including nurseries, childminders and Sure Start programmes. Since schools work only with children over three years old, this framework is confined to childcare services. After FS, from the age of six children become subject to yet

> ### Box 3.3: An example of nursery education grant in a private day nursery
>
> St James's is a private day nursery in a seaside town and started life in 1999. When visited, it had 38 places for children from babies to five years of age. It was open nine hours a day, 51 weeks a year. The owners had opened their first nursery in 1989 and ran two other nurseries in the same seaside town. In summer 2002, parents were charged £2.55 (€3.65) an hour for a child under two years, £2.30 (€3.29) for two-year-olds and £2.20 (€3.15) for three- four-year-olds. Pay for nursery workers was £5.10 (€7.30) an hour, with no pension or other benefits, which was the usual rate for the area.
>
> The nursery grant covered some of the costs of the three- and four-year-olds. There are two options: the grant is paid for two hours a day, five days a week for 33 weeks in the year, or for two hours a day, four days a week for 42 weeks. The owners opted for the second option, which still left 10 weeks a year uncovered by the grant. They reported that local families usually reduced their children's attendance during these unsubsidised periods. The nursery faced competition for three- and four-year-olds from other providers, notably local schools opening nursery classes. Most of the children who started at the nursery under the age of three years left at age three to go to local schools that parents preferred. The nursery then had to recruit other children to make up the numbers. This was putting the nursery under pressure, since the owners' policy was to subsidise the costs for children under two from the fees for three- and four-year-olds.

another regime, the National Curriculum. This does not, however, extend to school-age childcare provision. Indeed, for children over five years old in compulsory schooling, there is no curriculum or other sort of integrative framework covering both schools *and* childcare services, such as the FS provides for early education.

Children from birth to 18 years old, therefore, are liable to pass through three practice regimes, referred to respectively as a framework, a stage and a curriculum. In particular, two of these regimes appear to be in opposition to each other, embodying different approaches to education and understandings of learning. To many of our informants in the early years field, the FS represented a broad and child-centred approach, and stood as a defensive bulwark against the narrower, more didactic approach they felt was fostered in primary schooling by the National Curriculum. A leading figure in the early years field told us that:

> There is a huge void between children in primary school and other settings. A lot more work is needed so that those outside the early years sector know and understand how young children learn and what is appropriate and build on that in the bottom end of the primary school. I think it's a disaster. That

> was the main value of the FS saying this is three to five-year-olds, reception
> class children are in this and not the national curriculum.

In this case, some degree of horizontal integration achieved for three- to five-year-olds has not been matched by any vertical integration across, at least, early and middle childhood. While some (for example, the Early Years Curriculum Group) have called for extending the FS principles and practices up through primary school, it has proved hard, informants noted, to get teachers working with children over six years old interested in working with 'the FS approach'. That this is a major issue seems to have been recognised officially, with Ofsted carrying out a study in 2003-04 "into whether there is a clash between the play-based Foundation Stage and the more formal approach of the National Curriculum ... and whether the transition from the pre-school Foundation Stage to the National Curriculum, introduced in year one, is too abrupt" (Mercer, 2003, p 4). The government, too, shows signs of recognising the issue, with the appointment in September 2003 of the first-ever national director of the FS. One of the director's tasks is to work on the link between the FS and the first years of formal education in primary school, to try to achieve a more 'joined-up' approach between the FS and Key Stage 1 of the National Curriculum (Tweed, 2003).

Similar discontinuity – between early and later education – applies in the case of assessment. Currently all four- and five-year-olds must have a baseline assessment within seven weeks of starting reception class, with schools choosing an assessment scheme from over 90 accredited options. To streamline this, a general FS Profile was announced in September 2001. This approach aims to assess both children's progress towards the early learning goals and their learning needs. The assessment is accomplished through ongoing observation and assessment of a range of planned classroom activities, with each child's cumulative profile completed at the end of the reception year. The first cohort was profiled in summer 2003. The approach to assessment on the FS Profile is in strong contrast to the more formal approach of Standard Assessment Tests (SATs), used to evaluate seven-, 11- and 15-year-olds.

There are, however, signs that the government is reconsidering the appropriateness of the SATs approach for seven-year-olds. Under proposals announced in May 2003 (as part of a New Strategy for Primary Schools to enable 'every primary school to combine excellence in teaching with enjoyment of learning'), schools are to trial a new approach to assessment. More emphasis will be placed on teacher assessment and judgement, underpinned by tests but with some latitude in how and when they are performed.

Yet, despite the contrast between the FS and FS Profiles on the one hand, and the National Curriculum and SATs on the other, it is important to note (especially when it comes to comparison with Scotland and Sweden) just how prescriptive and centralised the whole English approach is. Dozens of learning goals are set down; the guidance to the FS runs to 125 pages; and FS profiling requires teachers to affix 117 labels to each four- or five-year-old under 13 headings. Wragg (2003, p 5), who is both a professor of education and a teacher of five-year-olds, comments that the FS Profile requires "reception class teachers to grade [each term a class of] five-year-olds by putting somewhere between 3,000 and 10,000 ticks and crosses in boxes".

Regulation

Since 2001, the regulation of schools and childcare has been integrated within Ofsted, childcare regulation having been transferred from local authority social services. As with administrative regulation, integration within an educational framework was not inevitable. The DfEE and DoH consulted and agreed on the need for a unitary regulatory regime. Integration in the National Care Standards Commission was therefore rejected, as it would have split childcare from education inspections (this would have been a problem as some childcare services deliver education).

Given the great number of childcare providers (including family daycarers), the integration of responsibility for regulation involved a large expansion of Ofsted, from 500 to 2,500 directly employed staff, and a whole new regional structure to administer this large task. This was a change of approach for Ofsted, which contracts out many school inspections, and had initially contracted out the inspection of early education services to a private contractor. At the same time as responsibility for inspection of childcare and education has been integrated, the work itself is situated within several different regulatory frameworks with different cycles, requirements and legislation (some educational, some relating to child welfare). Just for services providing early education or childcare, separate regulations cover: maintained nursery schools (inspected every six years); nursery education outside the maintained sector, that is, in childcare services (every two to four years); childcare services (every two years); and independent schools (every four years). Most recently, starting in 2003, the extension of tax credits to cover the employment of some carers working in children's own homes has introduced yet another regulatory framework, this time embedded in tax credit legislation.

As one informant involved in regulation put it, the situation is "a mess". One consequence is the problems caused for services such as Early Excellence Centres or Children's Centres, which seek to provide a broad and integrated approach incorporating education, care and other provisions and whose work spans different regulatory frameworks. In such cases, although inspections are carried out by one inspectorate, different pieces of the whole are covered by different regulatory frameworks: there is no single broad framework able to take a holistic approach to the work of a centre. While there is now widespread acceptance of the need to review and consolidate the whole field, so far no timing has been agreed for undertaking this task. Overall, therefore, integration of inspection has so far been partial: unified responsibility is combined with continuing divisions between childcare and education.

Services for children below compulsory school age

Departmental integration has not, as yet, transformed the pattern of services, which remain largely fragmented. Provision continues to be dominated by well-established types of services, each with its particular orientation and clientele: private day nurseries and childminders mostly in business to provide 'childcare for working parents', playgroups and schools mainly offering a part-time service with a more explicit emphasis on education and play. However, as Table 3.1 shows and we discuss later, there have been some shifts in numbers of places in different services, at least up to 2001: provision in private day nurseries and school-age childcare increased, while provision in playgroups and at childminders fell.

These trends have led to an ever-increasing role for private for-profit providers, and in particular for nurseries. By 2002, private businesses accounted by value for 86% of places in the UK 'nursery market', a higher proportion than in any other country, the remainder being accounted for by the voluntary and public sectors (Laing and Buisson, 2003); there are no separate figures for England and Scotland. Nurseries (together with homes for elderly people) have come to exemplify the liberal welfare regime's emphasis on private provision and market solutions, in which services are treated like any other private product for which there is a demand. What this process of marketisation means is captured in a recent news item on the acquisition of a Scottish-based nursery business by an English-based one:

> The purchase of Scotland's largest nursery operator eclipses previous consolidation activity experienced in the sector and makes Just Learning [the acquiring company] the second largest nursery operator in the UK ... now (offering) a total of 4,472 places across 56 places. The deal was financed partly by venture capital from its backers.... The company acquired Careshare in a move to expand the company's large-scale operations to the whole of Great Britain.... There are currently no plans to rebrand Careshare settings as Just Learning nurseries. (*Nursery Market News*, 2003, p 205)

The same report offers a wider view of market developments.

> It is thought that it will be at least three years before the whole of the UK reaches saturation point [for private nursery provision].... In many respects, the maturing of the nursery market mirrors that of the care home sector [for elderly people]. A period of expansion by organic growth in the early 1990s was fuelled by gaps in supply ... followed by large-scale acquisitions and mergers of major operators.... Analysts and providers agree that as a result of this process the market is likely to consolidate into five or six major chains over the next five years accounting for a larger percentage of market share. (*Nursery Market News*, 2003, p 206)

Table 3.1: Provision of childcare and early education services, England (1989-2001)

| | Childcare services (places) | | | | | | | School provision three- and four-year-olds (FTE) |
	Public day nurseries	Private day nurseries	Child-minders	Out-of-school care	Holiday play schemes	Playgroups	Total	
1989	28,789	46,589	186,356	NI	NI	409,063		
1993	21,400	112,400	300,700	24,600	80,500	396,900	936,500	491,250
1997	20,200	173,700	365,200	78,700	209,000	383,700	1,230,500	534,600
2001	18,200	266,100	304,600	152,800	598,000	330,200	1,669,900	537,150
% change 1989-93	−26	+141	unreliable	NI	NI	−3	NI	
% change 1993-97	−6	+54	+21	+220	+159	−3	+31	+9
% change 1997-2001	−10	+53	−17	+94	+186	−14	+36	+0.5
% change 1989-2001	−37	+471	unreliable	NI	NI	−19	NI	
Net change in places 1997-2001	−2,000	+92,400	−60,600	+74,100	+389,000	−53,500	+439,4000	+2,550
Net changes in places 1997-2001 (new series)				+167,417			+213,727	

Notes: Childcare services refers to registered places, whether occupied or not. School provision is based on pupils attending, expressed as full-time equivalents (FTEs) (for example, two part-time pupils count as one FTE).

The change in childminders between 1989 and 1993 is unreliable because of the introduction of new regulations under the 1989 Children Act.

Information on out-of-school clubs and holidays playschemes was first collected in 1992.

Sources: DoH, 1997; DfES, 2001; new series of local authority returns to DfES for 1997-2001 (unpublished; figures supplied by the DfES)

Against this wider background of continuing fragmentation, government has made some moves to stimulate more integrated forms of provision. The Early Excellence Centre programme was intended to develop, demonstrate and disseminate models of excellence in the delivery of centre-based, integrated multi-agency services for children, families and the wider community. These centres are supposed, therefore, to demonstrate services working in an integrated manner. While the programme includes some innovative and important examples of how an integrated service might look, in practice Early Excellence Centres remain the exception rather than the rule: moreover, they often result from 'early excellence' status being given to existing integrated services rather than the creation of new ones. In January 2002 there were just 52 centres (with 100 proposed for 2004), compared with literally tens of thousands of individual 'non-integrated' services such as nurseries, playgroups and nursery classes.

There have, however, been recent moves to create more integrated provision. The Neighbourhood Nurseries initiative, announced early in 2001, was intended to support children and families in disadvantaged areas by helping to fund well-designed premises in communities with little or no provision. The aim was for 900 nurseries, providing 45,000 'affordable childcare places' by 2004. These nurseries were mainly to be provided by the private sector, but with direct government funding, that is, supply subsidy.

The most recent and ambitious initiative is Children's Centres, first announced in 2002. The DfES has described them as "part of a plan to integrate local children's services". These centres "will bring together good quality childcare with early years education, family support and health services ... [also acting] as service hubs within the community for parents and providers of childcare services for children of all ages" (Cabinet Office Strategy Unit, 2002, p 4). An additional 'key service' required of all centres is assistance for parents moving into employment. The initiative is clearly targeted at poor families and communities, the aim being "to establish a children's centre in every one of the 20 per cent most disadvantaged wards" (Cabinet Office Strategy Unit, 2002, p 4) to reach 650,000 children under five years old by 2006. The first 32 designated Centres were announced by the DfES in June 2003, and in his budget statement in March 2004, the Chancellor set a target of 1,700 Children's Centres by 2008 (Brown, 2004).

Children's Centres will mainly be developed from existing provision, including Early Excellence Centres (the programme for which will end in 2004), new and planned Neighbourhood Nurseries, and existing Sure Start programmes. There may also be a place for schools, both nursery and primary. The Sure Start Unit is "very keen to see [nursery schools], where they are in disadvantaged areas, built upon to offer the full Children's Centre offer", while "extended schools may be particularly well placed to support the development of Children's Centres" (Sure Start Unit, 2003a, p 14).

Services for school-age children

Much 'extra-curricular' activity has been developing on school sites in recent years. Half of out-of-school clubs are currently based in schools. Additionally, a whole programme of Learning Activities or Study Support Services has developed, conducted out of school hours. The two areas – out-of-school care and study support – operate under different conditions, especially regarding funding (for example, parents pay for out-of-school care but not for study support), and are the responsibility of different parts of the DfES. These activities have, however, developed around the school and the school day rather than involving an integration with school or, indeed, any fundamental change to the organisation or running of the school. They have not been provided by schools and there is often little or no connection between the two types of services (see Box 3.4 for an example of school-based childcare from a study local authority). Indeed, childcare is often referred to as 'wraparound' or 'topping and tailing', both terms implying the centrality and separateness of the school day.

The new emphasis on extending the role of the school, discussed earlier in this chapter, may bring more changes. Not only will there be more school-based childcare provision and other services, some provided directly by schools, but it is also envisaged that some Children's Centres may be school-based (Sure Start Unit, 2003a). What is less clear, though, is how far the extended school concept will bring changes to the school itself, as opposed to an unchanged school acting as a site and resource for other services. It is noticeable that the government's childcare review (Cabinet Office Strategy Unit, 2002) refers on several occasions to 'integrating early years and childcare' and "opportunities to co-ordinate and integrate childcare and study support out of school", but no reference is made to changes in that part of the school dealing

---

Box 3.4: An example of school-based childcare

Primrose out-of-school club began life in 1994. It is open from 8am to 8.45am, then in the afternoons from 3pm to 6pm; it also provides all-day care in the holidays. It takes 28 children, parents paying £2 (€2.86) for a morning session and £6 (€8.58) for an afternoon session. In June 2002, the head of the club was earning £8 (€11.44) an hour for a 30-hour week, while assistants got between £4.50 (€6.44) and £5.50 (€7.87) an hour, with no pension or other benefits.

The centre is based in a primary school, which its children attend. However, it runs quite separately from the school, being a 'self-funded' charity managed by parents of children attending. Apart from the shared accommodation, for which the school charged a rent, there is little contact with the school itself. Two club staff also work as classroom assistants in the school, but these are quite separate jobs involving different employers.

---

with compulsory education. The same is true of the more recent Green Paper *Every child matters* (DfES, 2003a).

Staffing and training

The legacy of a divided system of services is matched by a workforce divided into three groups: childcare workers, educational or classroom assistants and teachers. All three groups are highly gendered, most of the work done by women, especially in the case of childcare workers and educational assistants. But whereas the latter two groups have low levels of training and pay, teachers are highly trained and considerably better paid. (See Table 3.2 for a comparison of these groups across a number of dimensions.)

Before 1997, not only were these groups distinguished by differing levels of training, pay and status, but the approach to training was fundamentally different. Childcare training took place through an industry-based organisation, the Early Years National Training Organisation (EYNTO), with a competency-based orientation: as one informant working in the training field put it, "National Organisational Standards are very good at teaching people to microwave steam clean a baby's bottle – but what they are not good at doing is saying to somebody this is how you deal with questions from a child who has just lost a grandparent – we don't equip early years workers to take a completely holistic approach to the care of children". In addition, there was a plethora of other national and local qualifications.

In sharp contrast, teaching was a graduate profession, with a single national qualification. The distinction between childcare and teaching was sustained through a split union structure, with different unions representing teachers and childcare workers (although union membership among childcare workers is low, especially in the majority private sector). The main teaching union restricts membership to graduate teachers and emphasises the superior position of

Table 3.2: Some features of childcare workers, educational assistants and teachers: UK (2001-02)

	% female	% under 25 years	% with NVQ Level III+	Average hourly pay (£)	% in profit sector
Childcare					
Workers (total)	97.5	26.3	36.2	5.12	62.8
Nursery workers	98.9	35.6	44.1	5.48	50.5
Childminders	97.7	20.6	27.1	4.14	88.5
Playgroup workers	94.0	16.4	36.0	5.13	41.8
Education					
Workers (total)	77.5	6.2	81.7	9.56	7.4
Teachers	71.6	5.4	97.3	11.07	7.2
Educational assistants	93.9	8.1	38.8	5.71	7.8

Source: Labour Force Survey, spring quarter 2001 and 2002. Analysis carried out by the Thomas Coram Research Unit. Data are Crown Copyright, used with permission

teachers within the care and education workforce. As the representative of a teacher trade union put it, "there is a role for other professionals working alongside a trained teacher, such as 'teacher assistants' ... they have a role but that is to support the classroom teacher".

Policy since 1997 has neither bridged nor questioned this basic divide: there are no signs of any movement towards a workforce integrating teaching and childcare. There remains a two-tier workforce, split between schools and childcare services but also existing within schools themselves. This gives rise to the situation found in one of our study local authorities, where nursery nurses provided early education with 'support' from six nursery teachers; yet the former were being paid far less despite doing (in their view) the same job as the teachers.

Rather than any moves towards the integration of occupations, attention has been paid to making it easier for childcare workers who want to move into teaching through a new form of Registered Teacher Programme specially designed for childcare workers. Priority has also been given to improving movement within childcare work. The many qualifications within the childcare sector have been rationalised: a qualifications framework, produced by the QCA and EYNTO (Qualifications and Training Framework for the Early Years) has reduced more than 1,500 qualifications into 20 groupings intended to facilitate progression through the different levels of NVQ. The intention of what is referred to as a 'climbing frame' of qualifications is, in the words of one of our informants, "to allow for both vertical and lateral career progression by all childcare workers including childminders ... (and) to encourage workers to progress through the sector".

In some respects the childcare and school assistant workforce has become more differentiated since 1997. Two examples illustrate this process. First, a new Foundation Degree for senior childcare practitioners has been introduced, opening up new career possibilities. Second, in April 2003 the government proposed a 'higher level' teaching assistant as part of its plan to remodel the school workforce and reduce teacher workload: according to the government consultation document, these assistants would be 'operating at a level of understanding and competence equivalent to NVQ Level IV' and among other tasks would free teachers to plan, prepare and assess away from the classroom. These proposals are made in the context of a large increase in the number of assistants in schools (see Box 3.5 for examples from one of our study local authorities). In both its 1998 and 2001 education Green Papers, the government set out its intention to increase the number of teaching assistants substantially: from 1996 to 2002, the numbers of teaching assistants and other non-teacher staff increased from 91,000 to 167,000 (ONS, 2003b, Table 3.24). This increase, as well as increasing demands from teachers for more 'non-contact' time, has led to greater attention being paid to defining the roles of these assistants, especially in relation to teachers.

> ### Box 3.5: Two examples of the widespread use of teaching assistants
>
> The headteacher of a primary school with 280 children aged four to eight years has increased the number of 'learning support assistants' (LSAs) so that now there is an LSA in each class, with two in the nursery class. For this she has made particular use of her special educational needs budget. LSAs work with all children, but devote part of their day to children with special education needs.
>
> The headteacher of a middle school in the same area, taking 278 children from eight to 12 years old, had 12 teachers and six LSAs, four of whom worked part-time. Six years ago, when he came to the school, there were only two LSAs. They mainly work with less able children, in particular in mathematics and English, but two do other activities, including counselling: coming into the work as parents of children at the school, they have now become very experienced and have developed their skills.

Integration at the local level

A number of authorities have relatively long-standing commitments to working in a more integrated way, reflected in departmental organisation and policies. More recently, some have gone further, seeking new relationships between education, childcare and social services. The three local authorities researched for the study illustrate the range of solutions. One had moved well down the integration road, with a new Children, Schools and Families Department incorporating a range of services including childcare, education and children's social work (see Box 3.6). The second authority retained separate education and social services departments. These two departments had made a joint senior appointment – a Head of Early Years and Childcare Strategy – although she was located in, and mainly worked with, education. Overall, there was little contact between education and social services, in particular because social services was seen as desperately stretched and able to deal with only very serious cases. The third authority had three divisions – Children's Services, Schools Services and Community Services – reporting to one director (Education, Community Services and Social Care). All three had some interest in childcare and early education services, for example with respect to nursery education and out-of-school care, which were provided by two and three of the divisions respectively.

Alongside these varying inter-departmental relations, determined by each local authority, the Labour government early on established a new local integrative mechanism. Starting life in 1997 as Early Years Development Partnerships, with the remit of delivering free part-time early education, they became Early Years Development and Childcare Partnerships in 1998 with the added remit of delivering the National Childcare Strategy. Although local

Box 3.6: Local reorganisation of children's services

One of our study local authorities was a large county in the south-east of England with a population of just over one million. In April 2001, the local authority had reorganised its services for children into a new department, named Children, Schools and Families. This was the culmination of two years of consultation and planning, during which the many cross-sector meetings had been, all informants said, successful in winning 'hearts and minds'. The department spanned a wide range of universal, targeted and special services. Universal services were open to anyone, although not all of them are universally provided; they include schools, childcare and youth services. Targeted services were aimed at particular children (for example, anger management support) or at particular areas (for example, Family Centres). Special services include adoption work, respite care and child welfare. The intention was that early intervention through universal and, less frequently, targeted services would support children and families, nip small problems in the bud, and lessen the need for special services.

The department was based on four areas or quadrants, each providing a multi-professional children's team, with services clustered around school communities.

These local teams consisted of: early years, community development and preventive workers; referral and assessment teams; educational welfare and educational psychology; and long-term work including looked-after children, child protection, family support and disability teams. The intention was to provide a unified casework service to children and families whose problems could not be dealt with by universal services alone, and to develop 'local preventative strategies' to prevent children failing at school or being brought up by parents who were insufficiently supported.

education authorities have ultimate responsibility for EYDCPs, the intention was to bring together a 'diverse range of providers covering early years and childcare, and to a lesser extent business, employment and regeneration interests' (Cabinet Office Strategy Unit, 2002, p 48).

Our informants had different views about them. One informant working in government described them as "bodies for consultation and representation ... [but] not in control of any aspect of policy delivery.... [They] are forums bringing people together but participants are not interested in the full agenda.... They're all fighting their own corner". This informant thought that, strategically, local authorities should take the lead in the partnerships – but that this would cause dissatisfaction and disruption among other members who would see their interests threatened. Another critical respondent, working with a voluntary organisation, referred to EYDCPs being "a huge task ... [as an organisation] we've always encouraged local forums and then partnerships. But never advocated that such an important service should be determined by a non accountable body. There is a problem around representativeness and workload". The lead office for the EYDCP in one of the study local authorities also referred to the heavy workload for members of the partnership (she herself was exhausted) and the reliance of women workers on short-term contracts (only three of 60 staff in her partnership had long-term contracts).

Somewhat contrary to this, another informant, an academic who also chaired a partnership, said EYDCPs generally worked well and were a move towards democratisation. They did, however, vary, with some dominated by their local authority (contrast this critical view of local authorities with the previous informant, who thought they should lead – both know that something is wrong but make different suggestions for putting it right).

Finally, the representative of a national organisation noted that education was proving the most difficult body to involve in local planning. This, she thought, would prove very problematic if there was to be a movement to make schools a central focus for a wide range of children's services. This was illustrated in one study authority in which schools were said not to be much involved with EYDCPs.

It was generally agreed that there was considerable variation in how well and in what ways EYDCPs work, 'from very good, through mediocre to terrible', as one informant, well placed to comment, put it. This has been acknowledged by government, the interdepartmental childcare review noting that only about a fifth of EYDCPs work well, and that "EYDCPs have often required intensive support from DfES as well as local authorities ... and that where they are working well it is because of clear leadership on the behalf of the LA" (Cabinet Office Strategy Unit, 2002, p 49). The review also concludes that "the message from the centre that EYDCPs are the local delivery agents has caused some confusion about what EYDCPs are expected to deliver and what they can actually do within the law" (Cabinet Office Strategy Unit, 2002, p 49).

The result appears to be a future sidelining of EYDCPs in favour of an enhanced role for the local authority. The childcare review concludes that "greater responsibility for the delivery of [childcare] services should be devolved to LAs" (Cabinet Office Strategy Unit, 2002, p 54). However, rather than locating this responsibility in the local education authority, the review favours placing responsibility for childcare in the Chief Executive's office, since "the childcare vision as a whole cannot be delivered narrowly through one arm of the LA such as the LEA, but needs to take account of cross-cutting local interests in health, social services, planning and regeneration as well as encompassing employment and local labour market interests" (Cabinet Office Strategy Unit, 2002, p 53).

Just as, at national level, emphasis has been placed on childcare as a means to many policy ends, which justifies its removal from an exclusively educational responsibility in departmental terms to a shared responsibility, so too this rationale is pointing towards childcare being placed outside an educational setting at local level. Once again, this reveals how central government views 'childcare' as a distinct field with a relationship with education among other policy fields, rather than being inseparably and specially connected with education.

Relations with other services

As already noted, developments in the relationship between childcare and education need to be seen against the government's wider policy agenda, in particular the development of a Children's Strategy, with a unit having responsibility for overseeing the strategy. This reflects the Labour government's emphasis on 'joined-up working', crossing departments, with general mechanisms such as cross-cutting reviews and the Comprehensive Spending Review intended to focus departmental minds on common concerns and outcomes. But what implications did the transfer of responsibility of childcare from welfare to education have for relations between the two areas of government most involved with children and young people – the DfES and the DoH?

The transfer of childcare to DfEE left the DoH with responsibility for relatively small groups of children and young people, in particular those in need, at risk or looked after, as well as a responsibility for the health of all children. The DoH embarked on a range of policy developments mainly concerned with these areas of responsibility. It undertook the development of a National Service Framework for Children, intended to provide a 'performance management framework for children's services' or, more specifically, services for which DoH still had responsibility, that is, not including schooling and childcare services.

In October 2002, the Secretary of State at the DoH announced his intention to create specialist Children's Trusts bringing together a range of agencies including social services, health and education. The role of these trusts was to jointly plan, commission, finance and sometimes deliver services, their aim, according to the DoH website, being "to ensure children and their parents get better coordinated services geared to meeting individual needs". At the same time he referred to plans to develop new types of occupations, including "family care workers combining the skills of the health visitor and the social worker to provide family support in times of trouble" (Milburn, 2002).

These plans for Children's Trusts and new types of occupations have been somewhat overtaken by events, which have further marginalised the position of the DoH with respect to children. In June 2003, the government decided to appoint a Minister for Children, Young People and Families, and located this post in the DfES, the department that already had responsibility for most children's services. This new post was given responsibility for a wide range of services, working through a new Children, Young Peoples and Families Directorate. Some of these services were already in DfES (including the new Sure Start Unit, the Connexions mentoring and career guidance service for 13- to 18-year-olds, special education needs and the youth service). But other services were transferred from other departments, including family and parenting law and support (from the Lord Chancellor's Department), the Family Policy Unit (from the Home Office) and child welfare from the DoH. So, having been a key player in children's services in the early 1990s when the 1989 Children Act was being implemented, within a decade the DoH has lost nearly all non-health responsibilities for children.

One feature of these most recent changes should be highlighted as particularly significant to our enquiry into the relationship between early years education, compulsory schooling and 'childcare' services. A press release from the DfES describes the new arrangements in the following way:

> ... the integration of children's policy into DfES will create a single departmental focus for children, including disadvantaged children, improved coordination within children's services (including family and parenting support), *and between these services and mainstream schools and education policy.* (DfES, 2003a; emphasis added)

The new Minister for Children may have responsibility for a wide range of children's services, including 'childcare' and early years education, but her remit does not include the most central service of all: schools. There is, it appears, 'children's policy' and there is 'mainstream schools and education policy'. Rather than integration, childcare, early years and compulsory education need 'improved coordination'.

Similarly, the idea of new occupations has disappeared from the agenda. The government's Green Paper following this major departmental reorganisation envisages common occupational standards across work with children linked to modular qualifications, with no reference to new occupations or professions. The proposed Children's Workforce Unit will not include teachers, but will "work closely alongside the existing School Workforce Unit" (DfES, 2003a, para 6.49), implying a continuing split between, for example, childcare workers and teachers.

Locally, plans for pilot Children's Trusts in selected areas have now been superseded. The Green Paper envisages early legislation requiring all local authorities to appoint a Director of Children's Services, to be accountable for education and social services. But the government's "longer term vision is to integrate key services within a single organisational focus". Its preferred model is Children's Trusts, expected to be in most areas by 2006. 'Key services' that should be within these trusts include the local education authority, potentially covering all education functions including childcare, early years education and school improvement; children's social services; and community and acute health services. But additional services might also be part of a trust, such as youth offending teams and the Connexions service (DfES, 2003a, paras 5.12-5.14).

The differences at local level between our three study local authorities in the degree to which services and departments were being integrated is likely, therefore, to reduce dramatically in the future, as all move towards the integration of 'key services within a single organisational focus'.

Observations

Integration of departmental responsibility for early childhood education and care services, schooling and school-age childcare has taken place against the background of a wider programme of change affecting policy and services for children. There have been new structures, new strategies and programmes, new systems for control and regulation, and new money. Increased attention has been paid to closer and better-coordinated relationships between departments offering a more 'joined-up' approach to particular policy priorities, culminating in a Minister for Children with responsibility for most children's services – except for compulsory schooling and child health. New policies and services reflect new policy aims, notably a strong commitment to eradicate child poverty and to increase the numbers of employed mothers, especially lone mothers; and, in support of these aims, a clear commitment to support employed parents, including the development of 'childcare' services that are generally available and accessible.

These changes have been driven by a strong and active national government, with HM Treasury seeking to apply some coherence across policies in order to focus them on what it considers to be vital domestic policy goals – eradicating poverty and social exclusion, increasing employment, enhancing competitiveness. Social policy in fields such as childcare and education has been formulated and implemented through an extraordinary degree of central direction and regulation, by either government departments or government agencies, reflected in an immense weight of documents distributed downwards setting out how policy should be implemented, and controls that attempt to ensure delivery and compliance.

What has been lacking is much sense of reflection on basics, including principles, concepts and structures: constant action has left little space for thought and debate. Difficult issues – for example, those thrown up by consideration of the workforce involved in working with children – have not been confronted; assumptions – for example, that 'childcare' is a distinct field and normally a private responsibility – have been insufficiently questioned; new approaches to services, like Children's Centres, have come late in the day and have been partially applied; options have not been set out publicly, so stifling any climate of discussion; consultation questions in departmental documents often take a narrowly technical form – for example, the CCTC was introduced as a main form of funding without any review or consultation about different funding methods or, indeed, about the sharing of costs between families, employers and state.

Despite this, policy developments in the early education and childcare fields have not met much opposition, politically or professionally. Indeed, given the great importance that government has attached to these fields, they have generated remarkably little political debate, and were almost invisible in the 2001 election campaign. Moreover, while there may have been some doubts about details of policy, some disgruntlement at the workload passed down from government and some confusion over the sheer number of different initiatives, most people and organisations involved in early years and childcare have recognised that the Labour government has brought a new policy interest to the field, backed by additional resources. They have been prepared to do their best to respond to the demands made upon them.

From our interviews we obtained a clear sense of a break with the past. The 1997 election marked a new era in a previously neglected field, not least because government has for the first time in peacetime given recognition to the importance of childcare (the importance of early education had been recognised by the previous Conservative administration). As one informant from a voluntary organisation put it, "We've seen an unimaginable change in four years".

At the same time there are striking continuities in policy and provision with earlier administrations. We shall consider the extent of the process of integration in England – between early childhood education and care, schooling and school-age childcare – in comparison with Scotland and Sweden in Chapter Six. For the moment, we would characterise the process as limited: for example, 'childcare' is still widely understood and spoken of as a distinct field. Symptomatically, government has had an interdepartmental *childcare* review, intended to 'develop a vision for 2010 for *childcare* in England', and which refers to *childcare* services and *childcare* providers, the *childcare* workforce and the *Childcare Tax Credit*; the Chancellor has since announced a further review of *childcare* policies to inform the next Comprehensive Spending Review.

There are other continuities which can perhaps best be understood in relation to some of the context features discussed in Chapter Two, in particular the continuation across administrations of an essentially liberal welfare regime. For both practical and ideological reasons, the Labour government has often worked with the existing system, not least as the best and most expeditious means to deliver the extra childcare places so urgently demanded. The 2002 interdepartmental childcare review, for example, is an essentially technical document focused on how to improve the workings of the existing system, taking the main features of that system for granted, not a critical examination of that system and its attendant assumptions and structures.

Much post-1997 policy, therefore, has involved building on what already exists and working with well-established principles. We can take five examples of such continuity. First, *market approaches* have been confirmed, indeed reinforced, as has the dominant position of private for-profit providers in what is still thought of and referred to as the 'childcare' sector. Childcare services are provided largely through the private sector, with parents expected to select and purchase the product that suits them best: this is the hallmark of the advanced liberal state, which expects citizens to assume responsibility for their own risks. At the same time, the previous Conservative government policy on early education has continued: funding supports a market that offers the possibility of choice between a range of services and the public and private sector (although the actual means of funding was changed with the dropping of vouchers).

The 2002 interdepartmental childcare review is replete with the language of the market: there are "shortages in most childcare markets"; "the primary mechanism for delivering new [childcare] places is through pump priming to encourage childcare business start ups"; "more needs to be done to address areas of market failure"; "branding is confusing parents"; "the spending review provided funding to support the Government's vision of a childcare market where every parent can access affordable good quality childcare". Government interventions, such as CCTC and neighbourhood nurseries, are justified in terms of 'market failures', in particular those arising from difficulties experienced by low-income families in accessing services in the private, unmediated market. In effect, the long-established policy principle that childcare is a private responsibility of parents, with a role for government in regulating the market, remains in place: what has changed are the details of policy, in particular public policy playing a more active role in stimulating supply (through expanding on the small initiative of the previous Conservative government to provide short-term 'pump-priming' funding) and increasing the ability of lower-income families to afford private services (again building on a smaller-scale initiative of the previous government).

A final element in this continuity of approach emphasising the private nature of childcare services is the continuing hope that individual employers will support childcare for some of their employees as part of a package of employment benefits. The English National Childcare Strategy asserted that employers "have a vital role to play in delivering the strategy" (DfEE, 1998), while the recent childcare review argues that "employers could do more to help with childcare" (Cabinet Office Strategy Unit, 2002, p 22). The review goes on to say that government "will continue to promote the business case for various forms of childcare assistance" (Cabinet Office Strategy Unit, 2002, p 27). Nothing illustrates more clearly the continuity in policy development and the attendant lack of reflection than this persistent quest for an 'employer role', despite its failure in practice – employers are estimated to contribute 6.5% of total day nursery costs (Laing and Buisson, 2003) – and the contestability of the principle (Moss, 2001).

Second, while there is often a rhetoric of universality, government policy in practice maintains a strong element of *targeting*, one of the hallmarks of a liberal welfare regime: for example, most of the main post-1997 initiatives in the 'childcare' field are targeted. Sure Start, Neighbourhood Nurseries, Children's Centres and full-service extended schools are all aimed at disadvantaged areas, CCTC at lower-income families. Most parents in most areas therefore will not benefit. Indeed, what is emerging is a two-stream approach to services: a new generation of government-funded integrated services in a minority of poor areas, and a private market of 'old generation', fragmented services elsewhere. The only exception to this form of targeting is the provision of early years education, which is established as a universal entitlement – although even this entitlement is targeted at a particular and narrow age group, three- and four-year-olds. It is perhaps significant that the single unit that emerged after the 2002 Comprehensive Spending Review – responsible for early education, childcare services and the Sure Start programme – was called the Sure Start Unit, adopting the name of a targeted initiative.

Third, we can see strong continuities in *the structure and regulation of education*. Early education has retained its part-time basis, a policy going back to the Plowden Report of the 1960s (Central Advisory Council for Education, 1967). The FS covers a three-year period of education for children from three to five years of age, but compulsory school age remains five years, and many children still start primary school at four years of age. The organisation of compulsory schooling itself has been left untouched by the advent of more childcare and other activities for school-age children, which remain 'out of school' or 'wraparound'. More broadly, the pre-1997 trend in education towards an evaluative state and quasi-markets has been sustained.

Fourth, despite the priority attached to childcare and early education, there does not appear to have been a noticeable acceleration in the rate of *increase of services*, at least if one compares the last four years of the Conservative administration with the first four of the current Labour administration (see Table 3.1). Levels of provision between 1993 and 2001 reveal no sudden surge after 1997. For example, places in private day nurseries increased by 54% between 1993 and 1997, and by 53% between 1997 and 2001, while places at childminders increased by 21% before 1997 and fell 17% in the following four years. Numbers of three- and four-year-olds in school rose 9% between 1993 and 1997, but were static from 1997 to 2001. If we look at government statistics for three- four-year-olds receiving early years education (in schools or private sector services) over the period 2000-03, the increase in numbers is modest (up 4.6%): the change is in the proportion of children whose places are publicly funded, which has grown from 71% to 96% (ONS, 2003a, Table 1).

Various qualifications need to be made, meaning that our or any other conclusion must be treated with great caution. First, the lower the baseline (as it was in 1993 compared with 1997), the easier it is to show rapid growth rates and the harder it is to sustain them over time. Second, government policy may have taken time to have effect after 1997. Finally, the statistics omit important developments such as Sure Start programmes. As we have already noted earlier in this chapter, there are also problems with the statistical sources themselves: the source that enables pre- and post-1997 comparisons ended in 2001; the government has used a different source for tracking post-1997 changes, but this source is not published, does not go back before 1997, and gives increases in places without also supplying data on the total number of places available. Moreover, as Table 3.1, shows there are large discrepancies between the two sources for the increase of places between 1997 and 2001: they give very different results. Yet a third source has been introduced from 2003, but this is not comparable with the other two sources.

What both sources do agree on, however, is that most of the post-1997 net increase in places has been in school-age childcare services. In this important but relatively low-cost service, provision has grown substantially. For example, as Table 3.1 shows, these services account for just over three quarters of the net increase in places between 1997 and 2001. Even so, the rate of increase in these services between 1997 and 2001, combining out-of-school and holiday schemes, was very similar to that between 1993 and 1997.

A report of the National Audit Office (2004), published just as this book went to press, confirms a number of these conclusions. Between 1999-2003, 626,000 new childcare places were created in England. But over the same period 301,000 places closed – leaving a net increase over the four years of 325,000. Moreover, this net gain (70%) was in school-age childcare services, with a net gain of just 96,000 places for children under five. The numbers of three- and four-year-olds in schools hardly changed. The increase in this age group receiving funded early education was accounted for by children attending services in the private and voluntary sectors; many of these children would have attended these services already, the main change being that now part of their attendance time is funded by the nursery grant.

A final continuity concerns the major divides of policy and provision. *Integration between education and care and between early years and compulsory schooling has been limited.* We have already emphasised the conceptual and structural separation of childcare from education. But a similar divide continues between early years and compulsory education (at least from six years of age): indeed, this divide may have widened as either pressure on schools to improve educational standards or a particular view of standards has intensified. Several informants spoke vehemently and at length about "a clear divide between people who have an early years perspective and a primary and secondary perspective". Another, a researcher, spoke of "a mismatch in government strategy for early years and primary. The government says children and families need an integrated service, a holistic view and then suddenly they go to school and all that stops, it's about academic performance". Yet a third described how recent changes in compulsory schooling were making the teacher's relationship with children narrower and more instrumental:

> "Schools have been under pressure and it's made more of a distance from the children.... The timetable is very dominating, it undermines continuity, the pressure is on the objective for today and how to achieve. It is a very important role to build social and emotional relations with children, but there is far more attention to the objectives. I left teaching myself when the National Curriculum came in because it is very objective-led, attainment targets, and I could not go off and talk about new schools with a five-year-old."

Just as differing government aims were pulling care apart from education, so different policy agendas were widening the gap between early education and compulsory education. One experienced observer recounted, using metaphors of warfare, that "the biggest battles I've seen are between the DfEE and Ofsted and the National Literacy strategy – the fight for reception [class children] and it's still going on.... The battleground is the misunderstanding among those working with older children about what are appropriate strategies for those working with younger children".

Thus, bringing services together within the same department was no guarantee of conceptual integration across the three services on which we have focused. Rather, even within the same department, differences remained and festered. Fundamentally different ideas about childhood, learning and the school's role of care produced fundamental differences of policy and practice.

FOUR

Scotland

Emma's story

Emma was born in 1996 and, when this book was written in 2003, she was seven-years-old. She lives with her mother (Anne), her father (Mike) and older sister (Julia) in a village in the north of Scotland with a population of just under 1,000. She currently attends the local primary school where she is in her third year of compulsory schooling.

Emma's care and education, from birth to seven years

Mike works at the local fishery, which can involve long hours, Anne works full time at the village library. They are not well off, but they describe themselves as 'comfortable'. Mike's salary of £18,500 (€26,455) per annum is below the national average of £22,204 (€31,752). Anne earns £12,000 (€17,160 per annum) working full-time as a librarian assistant. This income is supplemented by the UK-wide universal Child Benefit, and with two children this works out as an annual amount of £1,393.60 (€1,993). Because of the level of their joint income, the family is not entitled to either the WFTC or the CCTC.

At the age of seven, Emma has already experienced a number of different care and education services. For the first two years of her life, she stayed at home. Initially, she was cared for by her mother, who had left the labour market after Julia was born. However, Anne decided to go back to work part time when Emma was around six months old, so her grandmother, who lived in the same village, looked after her and her sister Julia in the mornings while Anne worked.

When Emma was two years old her mother decided to return to working full time at the library and felt it would be unfair to rely on Emma's grandmother for the whole day. Instead, they agreed that Emma would go into a private day nursery in the mornings. (The nursery had opened only a year before, and Anne knew that they were lucky to get a place as daycare provision in rural areas can be difficult to secure.) In the afternoons, Emma would be looked after by her grandmother, as would Julia, now five, who had started compulsory school that year.

There were eight staff at the nursery (one nursery manager, one nursery teacher, six nursery assistants and a childcare trainee) who cared for around 35 children between the ages of two and five. The nursery assistants each earned £4.70 (€6.72) an hour, just over the national minimum wage; as most staff worked a 30-hour week, annual salaries were low, around £7,330 (€10,482) per annum, equivalent to about 30% of average earnings in Scotland. The assistants were all women between the ages of 18 and 24. The childcare trainee was working towards the Scottish Vocational Qualification (SVQ) in Early Years Care and Education (rather similar to the English NVQ) and was paid less than the assistants, £3.70 (€5.29) per hour. The nursery teacher, in charge of the childcare sessions for the older children, received £5.30 (€7.58) per hour, while the manager herself earned an annual salary of £17, 000 (€24,310).

All the assistants had specific qualifications in working with young children (SVQ in Early Years Care and Education, or Playwork or Higher National Certificates in Childcare and Education, mostly at Level II). Only the manager and nursery teacher had a teaching qualification.

When Emma arrived at the nursery at the age of two in 1998, her parents had to pay £2 (€2.86) an hour. As Emma tended to arrive early to attend the breakfast club (between 8am and 9am) so that her mother could get to work, her normal session lasted four hours at a cost of £8 (€11.44) per day. However, when Emma was three her parents were able to make use of the recently introduced pre-school education grant, whereby each day two hours of education were provided free of charge. This substantially reduced the cost to the family.

The pre-school education that Emma received for these 12 hours a week lasted two years – from ages three to five – and was provided in line with the recently published Scottish pre-school curriculum, which places a strong emphasis on play and learning through play. Topics covered include: emotional, personal and social development; knowledge and understanding of the world; communication and language; expressive and aesthetic development; physical development and movemen; and information communication technology. Emma stayed at the nursery until she was five-years-old and started her compulsory schooling.

Emma's care and education today, at seven years old

Now, Emma attends the local primary school, which is about five minutes' drive from the family's house. Emma is lucky that she lives so close to the school; many of her friends have to travel more than half an hour to get to school, some of them taking the small school bus. Emma's school day begins early when her mum drops her and her sister Julia at the primary school at 8am. Between 8am and 9am Emma attends the breakfast club, staffed by out-of-school care staff who are employed by a group of parents that runs the club with help from the local council's community education department. The club provides breakfast and charges £1.25 (€1.79) per day. The breakfast club is part of the new Health Promoting Schools initiative, in which Emma's school is involved along with a number of other schools in the area. Many of Emma's friends and classmates attend the club, so she spends most of her time there chatting and playing.

When the bell rings for the start of school at 9am, children line up behind their teacher and are escorted into the classroom. The primary school itself is small, with only 100 pupils, and around 40 of them come from the surrounding area rather than the village itself. The class teacher has a postgraduate qualification in primary school education. The class also has two part-time classroom assistants. One of these assistants, Carol, provides support to Emma's friend Paul, who has additional support needs. Carol used to work in the local post office, but decided to change jobs and took a short 'taster' course in childcare run by the local college (in a nearby town). The other classroom assistant, Michelle, provides much more general help to the class teacher, such as preparing and clearing up activities. Michelle had been a childminder but became a classroom assistant in order to gain additional skills, and is considering eventually taking professional training. The class teacher earns a salary of around £23, 000 (€32,890) per annum while the classroom assistants earn the minimum wage of £4.20 (€6.00) per hour.

Emma is taught in a class of 15, which, as part of a small village school, is far below the national average for pupils per class (which was 24 in 2000). During the day the pupils focus on the six key curriculum areas of language, mathematics, environmental studies, expressive arts, religious and moral education, and personal and social development and health education. These subjects are taught in a variety of ways, including individual, group and class teaching, and work from first-hand experiences, from books and from the blackboard. The subjects are taught in line with national guidance, although this does not constitute a 'formal' curriculum but allows teachers flexibility to develop their own learning and teaching plans.

Emma has just been tested on her progress in English (reading and writing) and mathematics, as it is expected that children will reach a basic level – Level B in the curriculum guidance – by the end of their third year at primary school. Emma's test was carried out by her class teacher and included a number of short exercises, completed as part of her normal activities at school. These tests are used to monitor progress and, unlike in England, do not contribute to national league tables of children's performance.

There is one break in the middle of the morning, when the children can play outside for 15 minutes. Some of them bring snacks such as crisps or apples to eat during this time. Lunchtime is from noon to 1.15pm and, unlike at the private nursery, teachers and pupils eat separately. The school meals are provided by catering staff and involve a choice of meals, including a vegetarian option. The children queue up and are served their lunch by catering assistants, and the children then pay for their meals. Emma eats at a long table with her friends, though sometimes, in summer, she will take a packed lunch from home and eat it outside. After they have finished lunch, the children go outside to play in the playground. They are outside most of the year, except in very bad weather, and are supervised by classroom assistants and occasionally by teachers.

Emma finishes school at 3.15pm but, as this is several hours before her mum and dad get back from work, Emma and her sister are picked up from school by their grandmother, who takes them to their home. Sometimes when they get home Julia and Emma play together and sometimes they have a little homework to do. Anne, aware that looking after the girls five days a week is becoming a strain for their grandmother, has recently become involved in setting up an after-school club in the local primary school. But the group working on this will have to explore funding before the plans can progress further, and any scheme they get going will be very dependent on parents' fees.

Emma's future care and education, from seven to 12 years

Emma will spend another four years in the primary school, moving up through the classes and changing teacher at the start of every new school year in August. She will continue to work on the key learning areas and to be tested on these key areas by her class teacher. By the time she is in Primary 6 (aged 10 years), she will also be taught a modern language, usually French, and probably taught by a specialist teacher working on a peripatetic basis.

At the end of her seventh year at primary school, when Emma is around 12 years old, she will move to the local secondary school in a nearby town. This school has over 800 pupils and a large number of specialist teachers who deliver the curriculum in their subject areas. The school bus will come past the village every day, drive her and her classmates to the school and then take them home again at the end of the school day. The local secondary school has just become a community school and will include a range of services such as community learning, out-of-school care and a 'one-stop shop' for a number of key specialist services such as social work and health. The family is hoping that the community school will change the system of school transport. At present, children from the village are unable to attend after-school provision at the school because they have to come straight home on the school bus.

> During her third and fourth years at secondary school (14 to 16), Emma will study towards her Standard Grades, which are national examinations on subject areas. When her compulsory schooling ends at age 16, Emma will have to decide whether or not to stay on to complete the Higher Grade examinations needed for entry to university.

In Chapter Two, we saw that there are many similarities in the structural conditions shaping reforms in Scotland and England: high levels of child poverty in families with children; rapidly growing employment among women with young children but with some groups, including lone mothers, lagging behind; social policies emphasising private responsibility, targeted state intervention and the role of markets.

We also drew attention to a number of differences. Some of these were demographic: a lower population density in Scotland, far more extensive and diverse rural areas with a variety of indigenous cultural traditions and languages, but with lower fertility and out-migration rates threatening the existence of many rural communities. Other differences involved structures and institutions. We also noted that Scotland fits less comfortably than England into the liberal welfare regime by which we have characterised the UK as a whole.

Before we move on to consider the reform process in our three services, it is important to add a few comments about the political context of Scotland since 1997, in particular concerning devolution. Scotland has formed part of what is now known as the United Kingdom since 1707, when the Act of Union established the Westminster Parliament as the legislative body for England, Scotland, Wales and Ireland. In 1997 the new Labour government fulfilled its pledge to hold a referendum on establishing a Scottish Parliament with power to vary the income tax rate. Subsequently, in 1999 Scotland regained its own parliament, which has so far been dominated by a centre-left coalition. Even before devolution, Scotland had retained many of its own institutions, including education and legal systems. Most child welfare, education and support services for children had long operated under separate legislation, although this legislation could be changed only by the Westminster Parliament. Governmental responsibility for Scotland was exercised by the Secretary of State for Scotland, with civil servants based within the government department known as the Scottish Office.

The establishment of the Scottish Parliament allowed much more legislative time for children's issues; and its first term, from 1999 to 2003, saw a flurry of legislation and activities in this area. But it is important to note that many important policy areas are 'reserved' to the Westminster Parliament. Employment provisions for parents relating to the birth and care of children, family social security and taxation measures (with the exception of an as yet unused right retained by the Scottish Parliament to vary the income tax rate in either direction by 3%) and equality legislation covering sex, race and disability are all determined by the Westminster Parliament (Table 4.3, p 105).

The new parliament has offered greater opportunity for developing distinctive policies. But the period of reform has also been one in which Scotland has found itself politically closer to England than at any time for two decades; during this period Scottish voters returned a majority of Labour MPs to the UK Parliament at Westminster, while England returned a Conservative majority. Since 1997, Labour has formed the government at Westminster and, since 1999, has been the main party within the coalition leading the Scottish administration. Some initiatives developed in England that are not in 'reserved' areas continue to influence services and policies north of the border to a greater extent than might have been predicted. For example, although not a reserved matter, childcare qualifications are also now delivered within a UK framework, and Scotland is involved in a number of other UK-wide programmes. These include the Sure Start early intervention programme initiated by HM Treasury and the NOF programme, both described in Chapter Three. These have sat alongside the major changes that have been embarked upon through the new Scottish Parliament.

The background to reform: services and change before 1997

Education has long been important to Scotland – a source of pride from the 16th century, when Scotland had four universities to England's two, through the 18th century Scottish Enlightenment of David Hume, Adam Smith, Adam Ferguson, Thomas Reid, James Watt and others. In the 19th century, the 1872 Education (Scotland) Act was seen as formalising – and making compulsory – an already extensive national education system:

> This was believed to be both meritocratic and democratic, resting on a ladder of opportunity that ascended from the parish and burgh schools through to the universities, allowing able boys from the most humble background to rise to eminence simply on the basis of their own talent. In Scotland it was believed that social barriers did not obstruct the path to success of the 'lad o' pairts'. (Devine, 1999, p 389)

As Scotland began to industrialise, the needs of younger children had begun to attract the attention of some employers and, in 1816, what may be described as the world's first integrated school, nursery and out-of-school service opened at what is now the World Heritage site of New Lanark in Scotland.

Distinctions between pre-school and school-age children and between education and care were less clear in these early services. The 1872 Education (Scotland) Act, by setting the age of compulsory schooling at five to 13 years, began to firm up the boundaries. The 1918 Education (Scotland) Act empowered local authorities to establish nursery schools for children over two and under five years old for those "whose attendance at such a school is necessary or desirable for their healthy physical and mental development" (1918 Education [Scotland] Act, Ch 48, Part 8). Subsequently, the 1945 Education (Scotland)

Box 4.1: New Lanark Institution for the Formation of Character and Infant School

The Institution for the Formation of Character and Infant School opened in New Lanark in 1816. Robert Owen, a mill owner and social reformer, opened the school and infant school for his employees and their children. They were intended to provide educational and recreational facilities for the whole community, and the school building also housed a community kitchen and dining room. In the year they opened they took some 600 children from the age of 18 months to 12 years. Owen described in 1813 how the nursery would combine care with education and would also provide "a place of meeting for the children from five to ten years of age previous to and after school hours" (Cohen, 2002, p 18).

Act placed a duty on local authorities to provide 'adequate and efficient' nursery education for children aged from two to five in the form of nursery schools and nursery classes (as categories of primary education). Nursery school and classes were deemed adequate "if such provision is made at centres where sufficient children whose parents desire such education for them can be enrolled to form a school or class of a reasonable size"(1945 Education [Scotland] Act, Part I, Section 1:6). Services developed slowly but on a more extensive basis than in England as a result of fewer four-year-olds being admitted to the first class of the compulsory school.

Childcare provision developed separately, being originally the responsibility of health authorities and the health department within the Scottish Office. Following the 1968 Social Work (Scotland) Act, responsibility moved to the Social Work Services Group, which included in its remit a range of childcare services for pre-school children, such as day nurseries, childminders, playgroups and family support services. School-age childcare was at this time the responsibility of the Education Department. Over the years, the location of the group changed, moving between the Scottish Office Education Department, the Home and Health Department and, in 1997, the Home Department of the Scottish Office. The 1968 Act imposed on local authorities a general duty to promote social welfare and a specific requirement to help children requiring assistance "unequalled in other UK legislation" (Tisdall, 1997, p 12). It also included a provision for local authorities to fund voluntary services in support of this.

At local level, the services became the responsibility of the new social work departments. These were introduced following a review of Scotland's juvenile justice system chaired by Lord Kilbrandon. His report, published in 1964, had recommended the establishment of 'social education departments' within local education authorities, a recommendation that was not followed. Instead, the separation of pre-school daycare and school-age childcare services from nursery education and schools was confirmed by the 1968 Social Work (Scotland) Act.

However, in 1986 Scotland saw the first attempt in the UK to integrate education and care in services for young children at local authority level, when the then Strathclyde Regional Council (covering nearly half of all pre-school children in Scotland) launched its Pre-Fives Initiative, giving all pre-school education and childcare services to its Education Department.

The motivation behind the reorganisation, according to the former head of the Pre-Fives Unit, had been to combine nursery education with the care of vulnerable and excluded children:

> It was about combining nursery education with the care of vulnerable and excluded children.... But there was no agenda for working parents and childcare was regarded with ambivalence or denial. 'We're not here to help mothers go out to work' I was told by one prominent (male) councillor. (Penn, 2002, p 14)

The Strathclyde initiative had a major impact, focusing attention on the education/childcare divide. By the time of local government reorganisation in the early 1990s, a number of other regional councils were reviewing their services.

In 1994 the Local Government (Scotland) Act replaced a two-tier system of regional and district councils with a single, all-purpose authority that came into force in April 1996. It required the new authorities to prepare decentralisation plans for their areas and removed a statutory requirement introduced by the 1968 Social Work (Scotland) Act to have separate social work and education directors. Reorganisation was unpopular but offered opportunities for some of the new councils to rethink their organisation and committee structures. Seven of them did so by bringing together, in varying combinations, education, social work, housing, community and leisure services (Cohen and Hagan, 1997). Stirling Council was one of the local authorities

---

Box 4.2: Strathclyde Regional Council Pre-Fives Initiative, 1986-96

Launched in 1986, the initiative involved giving the council's Education Department responsibility for all pre-fives education and care. The services were managed by the Pre-Fives Committee, a sub-committee of the Education Committee. The radical Pre-Fives Unit, headed for a long time by the former director of a childcare lobbying organisation, sought to make nursery schools the basis of flexible integrated provision such as community nurseries, and tried to integrate the pay and conditions of teachers and other nursery workers. Its policy of integration was criticised by the then Secretary of State for Scotland and the authority received no support from the then Scottish Office in its attempt to overcome workforce issues and professional boundaries. Strathclyde Regional Council was abolished by the 1994 Local Government etc (Scotland) Act but its education-based approach was continued in 11 of the 12 authorities that succeeded it.

Box 4.3: Stirling Council Children's Committee and integrated services

Following local government reorganisation, which came into effect in 1996, the new Stirling Council established a Children's Committee covering services for children within Housing and Social Services and Education and Community Services, and subsequently, in 1999, established an integrated framework for children's services bringing together early years education, out-of-school care, compulsory education and social work functions for children.

that opted to rethink its committee structures, and established a Children's Committee.

The 1989 Children Act, as we have seen, overhauled child welfare legislation in England and also introduced a new regulatory framework for childcare services. These regulatory provisions were extended to cover Scotland when lack of legislative time in the Westminster Parliament delayed similar revisions to existing Scottish legislation. The 1989 Children Act laid down that services for children below the age of eight required regulation (there had previously been no age limit) and in other respects strengthened existing provisions. However, the concept of 'children in need' within the 1989 Children Act was later reflected in the 1995 Children (Scotland) Act. This introduced a narrower focus than the general duties to promote social welfare and the enabling provisions to help children requiring assistance that were contained within the 1968 Social Work (Scotland) Act (Tisdall, 1997).

The narrow focus on children in need was balanced by a wider concern for the need for more child-centred structures and planning, which informed debate over the 1995 Children (Scotland) Act. This was described by the then Secretary of State for Scotland as "founded on principles derived from the UN Convention on the Rights of the Child" (*Hansard*, 9 May 1995, col 51). It introduced a number of important provisions derived from the Convention, including due regard being given to a child's views, subject to age and maturity, and the welfare of children being paramount in determining any matters affecting them. The new Act also picked up on the concerns expressed in a review of childcare law, published in 1991 (Tisdall, 1997) over the need for better inter-agency working and it placed a statutory duty on local authorities to prepare, consult upon, publish and review plans for all relevant children's services.

The new provisions contained in these Acts drew attention to the role of local authorities as facilitators and regulators of services. At the same time, the late 1980s and 1990s saw the growing involvement of central government in determining the content of education first in schools and subsequently in pre-school education. As Wilkinson (2003, p 4) points out, unlike in England, where the government took the legislative route, in Scotland the Scottish Office Education Department 'adopted a more relaxed approach' through the use of guidelines, for example, the publications of HM Inspectors of Schools in

Scotland, *Performance indicators and self-evaluation for pre-school centres* (1996) and *Curriculum framework for children in their pre-school year* (1997).

A new-found interest in nursery education brought a further policy initiative. As in England, a scheme for expanding nursery education through offering vouchers to parents of four-year-olds to choose from a range of qualifying services was introduced on a pilot basis in Scotland in 1996.

During the same period, a number of initiatives were introduced, centred in particular on school-age childcare. The Scottish Office issued a circular encouraging local authorities to offer their premises for after-school and holiday playschemes, and, as in England, a funding programme was established to set up – but not sustain – school-age childcare services.

By 1997, key features in Scotland of the field of study included:

- *Split departmental responsibility* and separate legislative frameworks at national level between welfare (Social Work Services Group within the Home and Health Department of the Scottish Office, responsible for daycare and childcare services) and education (Scottish Education Department, responsible for nursery and compulsory schooling).
- *A fragmented body of services* divided between welfare and education with different types of services, including nursery schools and classes, playgroups, day nurseries, family daycare and nannies. While provided for different purposes (childcare, play opportunities) and families (working families, families 'in need'), their use was less clear-cut. Working parents often needed to make use of a mixture of services, such as part-time nursery education or playgroups plus childminding, or use unregulated areas of care such as that provided by nannies and relatives, including a child's older sibling. The distinction between services had become further obscured by the government's nursery voucher initiative, which essentially gave the name nursery education to all services that qualified for delivery of 'pre-school education'.
- *A split between education and welfare replicated in the workforce*, which, in addition to widely varying qualifications, pay and conditions, particularly between teachers and childcare workers, also included a growing number of other kinds of workers involved in school-age childcare services.
- *A powerful if frustrated legacy, at local authority level, of the integration of education and care for pre-fives children* derived from the Strathclyde Pre-Fives Initiative. This had fed into the majority of authorities that had taken over from Strathclyde after the reorganisation of local authorities into smaller units (as discussed earlier). But the Strathclyde experience had also raised the profile of early years issues in other authorities. There was the beginning of some wider restructuring of children's services within a small number of local authorities, following local government reorganisation and the introduction of the statutory duty of children's services planning by the 1995 Children (Scotland) Act.

- *Increasing involvement of government in early years services and policies,* for example, by encouraging the development of school-age childcare services, through a scheme to support start-up costs and by offering premises, and by seeking to expand part-time nursery education through a range of low-cost services in addition to existing school-based services.
- *Growing acceptance by local authorities of a role of regulating, rather than providing, services and an accompanying growth in privately run daycare.* Nursery provision increased by 24% between 1994 and 1997 (Table 4.1). Most of this increase was due to a growth in day nurseries combining education and care, which grew by 61% over this period compared with a 7% increase in education-only provision such as nursery schools and classes. (Such evidence as is available suggests that most of this increase is in private provision; Scottish Office, 1996.) Out-of-school care grew by 325% between 1994 and 1997, rising from 3,261 children to 13,877 children (Table 4.1).

The process of reform

Changes in the run-up to the new parliament

A new dimension in Scottish politics opened up following the 1997 UK General Election, when a Labour government with an enormous 'change' agenda swept to power. For Scotland, one of the biggest changes, initially, would be the re-establishment of the Scottish Parliament in July 1999.

The excitement generated by the rebirth of the Scottish Parliament created an atmosphere in "which all things seemed possible" (Cohen, 2003, p 237). Children and young people featured in discussion over the legislation and procedural planning, and the Consultative Steering Group set up to design structures and processes for the new parliament recommended that the parliament should have 'family-friendly' working hours and engage with children and young people:

> We believe that young people should be given every encouragement and opportunity to make their voice heard. (Consultative Steering Group, 1999, cited in Cohen, 2003, p 237)

Early childhood services were high on the agenda of the incoming administration. Departmental responsibility for childcare services was transferred to the Education Department of the Scottish Office. However, within education the responsibility for services was still split. Early education from the age of three fell within the remit of the Schools Group, while a separate unit, subsequently a division, had responsibility for pre-school childcare and school-age children. At this time, staff within the Scottish Office who were allocated to early years were still few in number and, pending the establishment of the

Table 4.1: Number of children attending care and education provision (1988-2002)

	Total nursery provision	Play-schemes	Childminders	Out-of-school care	Playgroups	Crèches	Family Centres	Total
			Scotland childcare and education statistics (988-2002)					
1988[a]	48,001.0	na	10,775.0	na	46,838.0	na	na	na
1994[b]	73,337.0	9,749.0	31,780.0[c]	3,261.0	43,791.0	6,703.0	4,929.0	173,550.0[d]
1997[e]	91,264.0	7,325.0	34,553.0[f]	13,877.0	45,883.0	16,655.0	4,222.0	213,779.0
2003[g]	120,418.0	5,341.0	22,561.0	28,840.0	20,061.0	10,604.0	18,356.0	226,181.0
Change 1988-94 (%)	52.8	na	194.9	na	−6.5	na	na	na
Change 1994-97(%)	24.0	−24.9	8.7	325.5	4.78	148.5	−14.36	23.2
Change 1997-2003 (%)	32.0	−27.0	−34.7	107.8	−6.3	− 36.3	334.8	5.8
Change 1988-2003 (%)	150.9	na	109.4	na	−57.2	na	na	na
Net change in places 1997-2003	29,154.0	−1,984.0	−11,992.0	14,963.0	−25,822.0	−6,051.0	14,134.0	12,402.0

Notes:

[a] Home care services, daycare establishments and daycare services, 1998 (published August 1989) and Provision for pre-school children (published October 1990).

[b] 'November 1994 survey of daycare/education provision for children in Scotland (published March 1996).

[c] This figure slightly underestimates provision due to a lack of information on playschemes for 1994.

[d] From Scottish Office (1996).

[e] From Social Work Daycare Services for Children in Scotland, November 1997 and Summary results of the 1997-98 school census (published June 1998). It did not include nursery schools/classes with returns for those submitted separately to the Scottish Office Education and Industry Department; there may therefore be double counting.

[f] No figures are available for childminders in 1997. These figures were collected in 1998, reported in the 2003 summary results of the 2003 survey of childminders.

[g] Summary results of the *2003 pre-school and daycare census* (published by the Scottish Executive, July 2003). Centres' self-selected categories of provision.

Table 4.2: Pre-school education and care services

	Nursery schools/ classes classed as educational establishments	Day nurseries	Total nursery provision (educational + day nurseries)
1988[a]	40,855.0	7,146.0	48,001.0
1994[b]	49,760.0	23,577.0	73,337.0
1997[c]	53,260.0	38,004.0	91,264.0
2003[d]	68,835.0	34,635.0	103,470.0
Change 1988-94 (%)	21.8	230.0	52.8
Change 1994-97 (%)	7.0	61.2	24.4
Change 1997-2003 (%)	29.2	−8.8	13.4
Change 1988-2003 (%)	68.5	384.0	115.5
Net change in places 1997-2003	15,575.0	−3,369.0	12,206.0

Notes:

[a] Home care services, daycare establishments and daycare services, 1998 (published August 1989) and Provision for pre-school children (published October 1990).

[b] November 1994 survey of daycare/education provision for children in Scotland (published March 1996).

[c] From Social Work Daycare Services for Children in Scotland, November 1997 and Summary results of the 1997-98 school census (published June 1998). It did not include nursery schools/classes with returns for those submitted separately to the Scottish Office Education and Industry Department; there may therefore be double counting.

[d] 2003 pre-school and daycare census (published by the Scottish Executive, September 2003).

parliament, the main planks of early years policy were being put into place by the UK government.

The Scottish Childcare Strategy was published in May 1998 at the same time as the National Childcare Strategy was published in England. *Meeting the childcare challenge: A childcare strategy for Scotland* (Scottish Office, 1998c) outlined the government's proposals for 'good quality, affordable childcare for children aged 0-14 in every neighbourhood' in the three areas of quality, affordability and accessibility.

The document introduced the concept of Childcare Partnerships 'building on' existing early years forums and bringing together local authorities with private and voluntary providers, schools, employers, health boards, parents and others in planning and developing services. The strategy set only one target for increasing the number of places: to ensure that all four-year-olds have access to a part-time pre-school place 'by this winter' and, in the longer term, extending similar opportunities to three-year-olds (Scottish Office, 1998c).

The Scottish Childcare Strategy differed from the English National Childcare Strategy in only a few respects. One difference related to the role of the Childcare Partnerships. The Scottish strategy envisaged a somewhat stronger role for local authorities within childcare partnerships:

> We believe that the responsibility for convening and supporting the partnership should most appropriately rest with the local authority. It is important, however, that partnerships are not seen as local authority bodies. (Scottish Office, 1998c)

A further difference lay in the establishment of a Scottish Childcare Board, chaired by the Minister for Education and Children, which during its short lifetime (1998-99) took on a significant advisory role. (In November 1999 it merged with an early years education forum to become the Scottish Early Education and Childcare Forum.)

While the national and Scottish childcare strategies were being developed, HM Treasury was extending its involvement in the early years area. In addition to the new Childcare Tax Credit heralded in the English and Scottish Childcare Strategy consultation documents, it was undertaking a major cross-cutting review of all provision for children aged up to seven years, to consider whether multiple causes of social exclusion could be more effectively tackled at the family and community level through a more integrated approach to services than the previous system based upon dividing responsibility between departments (Glass, 1999, p 257).

The review gave rise to the Sure Start programme which, as explained in Chapter Three, was intended to provide an inter-agency approach to promoting the personal growth and development of children aged up to three years. Initially, it was uncertain whether this HM Treasury-initiated programme would cover Scotland, and it was first established in Scotland under the (rather wordy) title of Expansion of Support for Families with Very Young Children. Subsequently, in 1999, it became known as Sure Start Scotland. In Scotland, as in England, the programme is targeted on areas of greatest need "before [children] have the opportunity of pre-school education" (Scottish Executive, 2001b).

Unlike in England, the Scottish Sure Start initiative funds projects through local authorities and services that do not have to be solely used for partnership arrangements between local authorities and other agencies (Scottish Executive, 2001c; Cunningham-Burley et al, 2002).

Many aspects of Scotland's early years policy were therefore broadly similar to those being developed in England. The focus on facilitating access to employment and the demand-led approach to stimulating the development of services through tax credits involved areas of policy and legislation that had always been a UK government responsibility and would remain reserved to Westminster. The Sure Start programme involved services that had always been a matter for the Scottish Office even before devolution; its introduction in Scotland almost certainly reflected the growing influence of HM Treasury. In addition, a number of other developments that might hitherto have been seen as matters for the Scottish Office, such as the establishment of National Training Organisations and the launch of a Childcare Information Service helpline, were undertaken on a UK-wide basis.

By contrast, education policies were, and in general remained, more distinctive.

In Chapter Three we described the changes that swept through the English education system following the 1986 Education Act. Scotland was not immune from these changes but, as we saw earlier, it experienced them in a less prescriptive form, with curriculum guidelines rather than legislation and, as a number of senior civil servants commented to us, with local authorities remaining the preferred providers of education services.

An early initiative by the Scottish Office, following the 1997 election, suggested that schools would be playing a major role under the new administration. A New Community Schools pilot programme initiated in 1998 reflected in the adjective added to its title earlier movements in Scotland to link schools more effectively with the communities they serve (although an alternative name had been 'full-service schools', one of the wave of American school/community initiatives we referred to in Chapter One). The programme drew on the vision of schools as institutions for delivering lifelong and community learning, a concept which, as Wilkinson (2003, p 22) points out, was central to the Third Way political system expounded by Anthony Giddens. It is also worth noting that lifelong learning had been the theme of an EU European Year and the subject of a major Scottish Office conference in 1996. However, the New Community Schools programme was also seen – and increasingly became part of – a wider social inclusion strategy intended to assist in developing a more child-centred and integrated approach to school education, family support and health education.

Changes following the re-establishment of the Scottish Parliament

The Scottish Parliament was re-established in July 1999 under an administration led by Scottish Labour and supported by the Scottish Liberal Democrats. The new parliament had a high proportion of women members (some 40% compared with 18% at Westminster) and introduced new practices and procedures into UK political life. It is also worth noting that a large number of members came into the new parliament from local government, bringing with them some knowledge of children's services and awareness of the issues raised during the passage of the 1995 Children (Scotland) Act and during local government reorganisation.

The Scottish Executive was the name given to what is in effect the government of Scotland within devolved areas. The post of Secretary of State for Scotland was retained to represent Scottish interests in reserved matters within the UK government and as 'the custodian' of the 1998 Scotland Act (Scotland Office, 2002). (The post was subsequently abolished in May 2003 with the responsibility for reserved matters for Scotland and Wales taken over by another Cabinet minister within the UK administration.)

Box 4.4: New Community Schools pilot programme

Launched in 1998, the pilot programme was intended to offer "a new approach to identifying and meeting the needs of every child by organising and focusing the services which support children and their families from their earliest years through their development and education" (Scottish Office, 1998b, p 2).

The then Secretary of State for Scotland, Donald Dewar, noted that the schools would be piloted in the first instance in areas "where the challenge is greatest. But the lessons learned will be of practical importance to all schools and to all having contact with young people" (Scottish Office, 1998b, p 1). The New Community Schools prospectus set out eight essential characteristics for the pilot programme:

1. a focus on all the needs of all pupils at the school;
2. engagement with families;
3. engagement with the wider community;
4. integrated provision of school education, informal as well as formal education, social work and health education and promotion services;
5. integrated management;
6. arrangements for the delivery of these services according to a set of integrated objectives and measurable outcomes;
7. commitment and leadership;
8. multidisciplinary training and staff development (Scottish Office, 1998b).

The programme developed to involve some 170 schools or institutions in 30 education authorities in Phase 1, the majority of which were clusters of schools. The interim evaluation of the programme found a substantial increase in joint ways of working involving: education, health and social work; increased engagement with young people in schools through pupil councils and other means; and evidence of increasing involvement with communities. It also identified considerable structural, cultural and professional barriers to multi-agency working (Sammons et al, 2002). The original pilot New Community Schools were located in areas of multiple deprivation. However, in June 2001, Jack McConnell, Minister for Education, announced that the Executive would be supporting councils to roll out the New Community Schools model across Scotland, ensuring that every school would be a 'New' Community School in Scotland by 2007.

Integration and the joined-up agenda at national level

The new administration brought an immediate strengthening of earlier moves towards an integrative agenda and 'joined-up' working. Both parties forming the ruling administration had promised a minister for children, young people and families (Children in Scotland, 1999). The new minister, Sam Galbraith,

Table 4.3: Matters devolved to the Scottish Parliament/reserved to Westminster

Devolved matters	Reserved matters
Agriculture, fisheries and forestry	The constitution
Economic development	Defence
Education	Foreign affairs
The environment	Electricity, coal, oil and gas
Food standards	Nuclear energy
Health	Employment
Housing	Financial and economic matters (with
Local government and planning	exception of right to vary tax rate up or
Social work	down by 3%)
Some transport policy, such as Scottish	Social security
ports and roads	Equality legislation
Tourism	

took the title Minister for Education, with children included within his responsibilities, and shortly afterwards called himself Minister for Children and Education. The Education Department was reorganised, and the Early Education and Childcare Division established with responsibility for all pre-fives education and childcare services, and school-age childcare. It also had the task of rolling out the Scottish Childcare Strategy. The new division was one element in a more radical restructuring of the department, which in effect integrated responsibilities for education, childcare, and child and family welfare within one department, called the Scottish Executive Education Department (SEED). This involved establishing a new Children and Young People's Group alongside the existing Schools Group and moving higher education to another department (Enterprise and Lifelong Learning). The new department also contained the Chief Social Work Inspector and children's social work (with other areas of social work located in the health and justice departments) and Her Majesty's Inspectorate of Education (HMIE), until the latter became an independent Executive Agency in April 2001. Subsequently, a further division was added: the Information Analysis and Communications Division brought together the previously separate statistical units with technical services, research and information technology to provide strategic analysis for the whole department.

The new head of the Children and Young People's Group, Gill Stewart, writing shortly after it had been established, described it as 'offering new opportunities for better integration of both policy and funding':

> This should mean better services on the ground – and continuity of service – for families, children and young people. It should mean a more fully integrated approach to the needs of children and young people in the critical early years of life, in the pre-school years of life and at the important transition

points as they move towards adulthood and independence.... The new group will sit alongside and work closely with the Schools Group. This reflects a crucially important principle: that what happens to young people in school and outside school is related and interdependent. (Stewart, 1999, p 3)

Stewart noted that, although SEED brought together a wide range of responsibilities, it would still be necessary "to forge close links with other parts of the Scottish Executive – with health including community care, housing, criminal justice, social inclusion, sport and the arts.... Equally important we will need to involve children and young people themselves" (Stewart, 1999, p 3).

The Social Inclusion Unit was another new arrival to the Scottish departmental structure. Established a few months prior to the devolved government of Scotland, known as the Scottish Executive, it had the general remit of developing and promoting social justice policy through the Executive, but saw itself as working largely through other government departments, influencing others through the setting of targets. In this sense, it potentially had a wider strategic role throughout the departments that comprise the Executive. It also had a number of specific strategic tasks, including providing the secretariat to a social inclusion network and a ministerial task force on poverty as well as linking with the UK National Action Plan on Social Inclusion and Poverty.

The new Children and Young People's Group and the Social Inclusion Unit formed part of a wider agenda of 'joining up' – that is, coordination and collaboration between agencies, which had also been strengthened by the new duty of local authorities to prepare and publish children's services plans. The minister, Sam Galbraith, had been involved in discussions of this provision within the 1995 Children (Scotland) Act when his party was in opposition. Speaking at the Annual Conference of the Association of Directors of Social

Figure 4.1: Scottish Executive Education Department in 1999

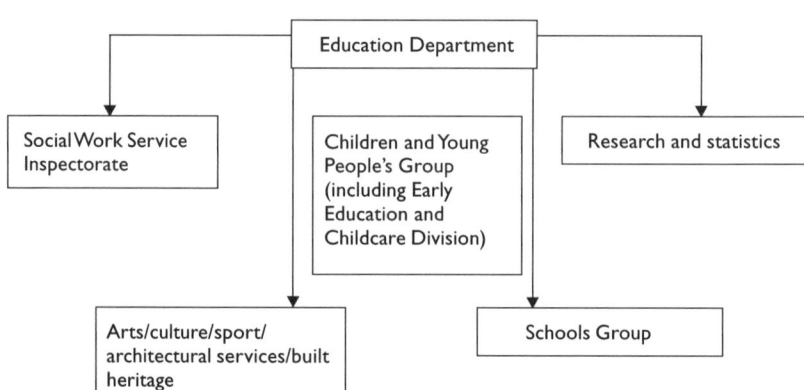

Work in May 1998, he expressed concern at "the lack of an overall framework for children's services" (Cohen, 1998, p 5). Subsequently, as we shall see, this wider integration agenda, taking in children's social services, was to become far more significant in Scotland than the integration of education and care.

What led to the restructuring of departments and ministerial responsibilities at this stage?

- *The cumulative effect of many years of advocacy.* As in England, many reports had advocated the need for an integrated, education-based, early years service.
- *The wider 'joined-up' agenda.* This was influenced by discussion around the enactment of the 1995 Children (Scotland) Act over the importance of planning across children's services and provision in the Act for a statutory duty on local authorities to prepare, consult on and publish children's services plans.
- *Extensive experience at a local authority level of education-based early years services.* Strathclyde Regional Council's education-based pre-fives services had covered nearly a half (47%) of under-fives in Scotland (GROS, 2001).
- *Increasing overlap between childcare and schools in early education.* The pilot nursery vouchers initiative had involved the delivery of early education in a range of childcare settings and brought increasing Scottish Office involvement in areas such as the curriculum.
- *The concept of social education.* The term was used in the 1968 Kilbrandon Report to describe social work functions and welfare activities that it had recommended should be located within education authorities. The Kilbrandon Report was formative in Scotland and was referred to by a number of interviewees, including some senior civil servants.
- *The 'modernising' government agenda.* The changes were seen by a number of interviewees as reflecting a move away from an institutionally driven agenda to closer community/customer/client-led objectives with a similar approach to services for older people – joining up policy initiatives around client interests and offering greater capacity to deliver on major cross-cutting issues.
- *Commitment and influence of a key politician.* The new Minister for Children and Education was seen by many of the civil servants interviewed as driving forward an integrative agenda. Sam Galbraith was one of a small number of Members of the Scottish Parliament (MSPs) who had also been an MP in the Westminster Parliament, where he is said to have coined the phrase 'joined-up working'. A respondent at a senior level within the Executive noted that both the change in ministerial title to incorporate children and the associated changes in departmental structures owed a lot to this particular minister:

> One of the factors in the changes had been the minister first appointed in the incoming executive. Sam Galbraith was experienced and had knowledge of children's issues.

- *The opportunity to restructure provided by a new institution.* The establishment of the Scottish Executive offered a further opportunity to revisit the structure of departments.

Further reorganisation had brought together responsibility for pre-fives education and childcare services and school-age childcare services within one division of the Education Department. The impact of the earlier Strathclyde initiative was clearly significant in this respect and was referred to by many of our interviewees. However, it did not seem to have clearly established, for those in government, what was required. As one senior civil servant told us:

> "The Strathclyde experience was not well understood in the Scottish Office. There was an awareness that there had been major impediments to the implementation of an integration agenda but not what they were."

Moreover, the main planks of childcare policy were already in place – and largely determined by a Westminster/HM Treasury-led agenda focused on facilitating access to employment and policy imperatives derived from the HM Treasury-led Cross-Departmental Review of Provision for Under-Eights. The opportunities presented by the location of the new group alongside the Schools Division were more constrained than was first thought.

Educational policy and the National Debate on Education

Within educational policy, the distinctive approach we noted earlier continued. The New Community Schools initiative was extended and, in 2002, the issue of the role of schools became the subject of wider discussion when the Scottish Executive initiated a national debate on education to consider what the education system of the future might look like. The debate asked:

- Why do we educate children and young people?
- What and when do children learn?
- How are learning and teaching delivered?
- Who can help this process?

An estimated 20,000 people took a direct part in the debate (Scottish Executive, 2002b, p 1).

Senior civil servants within SEED saw the debate as a ministerial initiative, stemming from international debate over the relevance of a long-established education model and echoing the questions posed in the report *Children, families and learning*, published in 1999 (Children in Scotland/Scottish Council Foundation, 1999). It was also seen as linking into the social justice debate.

The then Minister for Education and Young People saw the debate as a new way of developing policy through enabling discussion around services: "It is a new approach to policy development though people are struggling with it a bit as the notion of a genuinely open consultation is very new". The intention was to engage people in thinking "about how to develop a 'whole child' approach to education, on how other professionals might work in the schools and what children should be learning not just in an academic context but also in a broader social context".

An interim summary of the findings recorded not only well-supported views, such as the strong support for comprehensive education and for more pupil choice in the curriculum, but also explored a number of issues described as 'interesting ideas'. These included delaying the start of formal schooling until age six and adopting a 'continental' structure to the school day (Scottish Executive, 2002b).

The Scottish Executive's response to the National Debate on Education reasserted the Scottish Executive's commitment to comprehensive education: "I want to see excellent comprehensive schools at the heart of local communities" (Scottish Executive, 2003c, p 3).

The response refers to a desire for change:

> So people do want to see change. Above all they want a school system in Scotland that is well resourced and flexible enough to meet the needs of the individual child in a system that adapts to the child, not the child to the system. This will require radical new thinking about the way we design, build and manage our schools, about the way teachers teach, about the curriculum, and about the interaction between pupils, parents, community and school. It means making sure that all Scottish schools play a full part in lifelong learning. We must break down the barriers that get in the way of schools working flexibly with informal education, with further education colleges, with employers and with universities. (Scottish Executive, 2003c, p 4)

The Action Plan published by the Scottish Executive following the National Debate on Education provided for a three-year pilot on alternative structures to the school day with volunteer schools, and an increase in the opportunities for pupils to learn outwith normal school hours. It also sought to improve transitions from pre-five to primary schools, primary to secondary schools, and from secondary education to work or lifelong learning, and to enable teachers to work across primary and secondary schools.

School buildings and refurbishment programme

The possibility of change in education was further strengthened by a major school and nursery building programme funded through a public–private partnership programme. Projects worth over £1.15 billion (€1.31 billion) were announced in June 2002 and a further allocation of £110 million (€157.3 million) followed in February 2003. Scottish Executive ministers have sought to encourage "the most imaginative approach to design of our learning environment we can achieve" (Peter Peacock, Minister for Education and Young People quoted in Children in Scotland, 2003) and offers considerable opportunities to rethink relationships between schools, pre-school and school-age childcare services.

Every school to be an integrated community school

While these developments suggested the possibility of rethinking the relationship between schools and pre-fives and school-age childcare services, we found no evidence of any particular discussion along these lines; and the Scottish Executive's response to the National Debate on Education contains virtually no reference to pre-fives and school-age childcare sectors or any sense of where they fit within the overall vision that came out of the debate. The Coalition Partnership Agreement drawn up following the May 2003 election between Scottish Labour and Liberal Democrat Parties commits the administration to ensuring that by "2007 every school is an integrated community school", and emphasises "that these schools should be available to the whole community" (Scottish Executive, 2003a, p 25). However, it does not spell out in any detail what this might involve and does not suggest that any major changes are intended to current policies on pre-fives and school-age childcare provision to make schools a vehicle for developing greater vertical and horizontal integration.

The 'joining-up' agenda

Departmental restructuring does seem to have strengthened the moves to improve relationships between all children's services. As we have seen, the development of children's services plans introduced by the 1995 Children (Scotland) Act had highlighted the barriers to effective planning across child welfare, education, social care and health services. This was reinforced by the particular problems posed in addressing policy imperatives relating to child poverty, social inclusion and child protection. A number of interviewees thought that the new departmental structures had helped to address this issue. A team of experts from local government, the NHS and the voluntary sector was convened by Scottish Executive ministers to look at ways of better integrating children's services. The subsequent report, *For Scotland's children* (Scottish Executive, 2001a) concluded that services had often been badly coordinated and 'chaotic', with some children 'born to fail' and some invisible to services. The report, which drew attention to the problems created for services by an over-reliance on short-term project funding, proposed an action plan for achieving better integration at a local level. Significantly, the report argued that "despite their different history, boundaries and legislative requirements, children's services – encompassing education, child welfare, social work, health, leisure and recreation services for children from birth to 18 years – should consider themselves as a single unitary system". It also recommended that health should take the coordinating role for services for children under five, and education for children from five to 18 years. The report noted that health was implicitly the lead department for children under the age of five and recommended that this should be formalised with "the NHS taking the coordinating role for children before they enter formal education services and education fulfilling that role once children are at school" (Scottish Executive 2001a, p 90).

The response to *For Scotland's children* came from three Scottish Executive ministers and included an announcement of the establishment of a ministerial taskforce "to drive forward progress on integrated children's services"; the issuing of guidance on "taking a more integrated approach to planning children's services" (Scottish Executive, 2001d); and the publication of guidance on the use of the Changing Children's Services Fund (Scotland's share of the Children's Fund is described in Chapter Three). It was emphasised that this fund should be used as a 'catalyst for change' in Scotland, although focused on achieving better outcomes for vulnerable and deprived children "by improving sustainable solutions". Acknowledging issues raised in the report regarding the problems created by project funding, the response said that the fund should involve "improving the effectiveness and integration of mainstream services delivery" (Scottish Executive, 2001d).

The ministerial taskforce was later absorbed into a Cabinet Sub-Committee on children and young people, which in turn became the Cabinet Sub-Committee for Children's Services chaired by the Minister for Education and Children, serviced by the Children and Young People's Group with the First Minister as a member. A member of the group, which meets four times a year, described in an interview how the committee is intended 'to coordinate some of the work with children and young people'. The committee has focused primarily on developing the integrative agenda set by *For Scotland's children*, including integrated funding.

Box 4.5: *For Scotland's children*: action points for the integration of services

1. Consider children's services as a single service system;
2. establish a joint children's services plan;
3. ensure inclusive access to universal services;
4. coordinate needs assessment;
5. coordinate intervention;
6. target services. (Scottish Executive, 2001a, p 74)

The extent of integration at the national level

Departmental responsibility within Scotland

As we noted in earlier chapters, the starting point for our study has been the integration of departmental responsibility for childcare and education within the education system: what it has involved and what its impact has been. We have seen that, prior to devolution, an early decision was taken following the 1997 election to relocate responsibility for pre-school childcare services within the Education Department, where it remained divided from early education, the responsibility for which at this stage lay with the Schools Group. In 1999, following the establishment of the Scottish Parliament and the Scottish Executive, pre-school childcare, pre-school education and school-age childcare services were brought together within one division alongside the Schools Division and as part of a wider restructuring of the whole department. We found mixed views about what this had meant in practical terms. Among our interviewees some were sceptical that co-location within one department had overcome long-standing divisions between some areas of work, in particular as this related to schools:

> "The divisions within SEED don't talk to each other any more than the old departments did."

Since 1999, pre-school childcare and education and school-age childcare have constituted one division. However, we have noted that this area of policy has developed within the framework of a Westminster-led agenda. As a result there has been less room to take advantage of co-location in addressing areas of common interest such as qualifications and staff development. As we shall see later, the Early Education and Childcare Division has to spend a lot of time talking to colleagues elsewhere in the UK about how Sector Skills Councils take over from National Training Organisations, developments that do not (it is assumed) affect their education colleagues. Equally, the McCrone Inquiry on the pay and conditions of teachers (McCrone, 2001) was not asked to consider how this landmark deal might relate to the expanding workforce in early years and school-age childcare services.

Joined-up government

While the impact of bringing together departmental responsibilities has been less than might have been expected in respect of the early years policy area, it does seem to have contributed to wider aspirations for 'joining up'. A number of factors appear to have contributed to this.

First, as we saw earlier, the requirements at a local level to plan services on an interdepartmental and increasingly inter-agency basis, initiated by children's services plans and subsequently community plans, directed attention to wider coordination issues at a national as well as a local level. As we also saw earlier there has been a strong ministerial push to establish an overarching aim for children's services.

Second, the children's rights agenda was strengthened, as was visible in a number of early initiatives undertaken by the post-1997 administration, including, for example, the introduction of 'child impact statements' requiring all departments to consider the impact of any new policies on children. Once established, the Scottish Parliament promoted this agenda more extensively. More legislative time has enabled greater scrutiny, and coalition politics have altered the dynamics of legislation and committees. New education legislation has reflected wider support for placing greater emphasis on the views of children and young people and the parliament has also been afforded the space to examine other possibilities – notably, a Children's Commissioner.

Third, policies on social inclusion and child poverty, and the impact of a number of child abuse cases, drew attention to wider coordination issues.

However, of crucial significance in this wider 'joining-up' agenda has been the drive to 'modernise government' – described to us by interviewees within the Scottish Executive and Convention of Scottish Local Authorities variously as moving away from an institutionally driven agenda to community/customer/ client-led objectives, joining up policy initiatives around 'client' interests, and improving communication. At a national level, the then head of SEED talked to us of the organisational and cultural issues that needed to accompany any structural change.

> "Putting a structure in place is like putting up the walls of the house – it doesn't give you a functioning home."

He described some of the means that have been used to try to establish effective working relationships so as to bring individuals and groups together. Some interviewees were sceptical about what the structural changes had actually meant to date, noting that the department was still called 'education' and that the ministerial title had changed back again from Minister for Children and Education to Minister for Education and Young People, reflecting, it was suggested, the real priorities of the department. However, a number of interviewees were optimistic about long-term outcomes, suggesting that the process would take time. Joining up has certainly become a commonly expressed aim of many strategies – of which the draft *Integrated strategy for the early years* referred to in Chapter One is only one example. A number of vehicles are now in place to reinforce this approach, including a Cabinet Sub-Committee for Children's Services and the Office of Children's Commissioner. It is less clear how this can affect the education/childcare divide as long as childcare policy remains embedded within a largely Westminster-determined strategy.

Other areas of integration

Funding

Funding continues to be largely divided. As in England, the integration of care and education has gone furthest in funding pre-school education places across a range of daycare and play services as well as nursery schools and classes. The grant operates in a broadly similar way to England, funding places for all three- and four-year-olds for 2.5 hours, five times a week, in services that meet the specified criteria for offering pre-school education. The majority of places are provided within local authority schools. Over 80% of four-year-olds were in a council place in 1999-2000, compared with 15.4% in non-council-run services. The proportion is lower for three-year-olds with 47.6% compared with 26.6% respectively (Audit Scotland, 2001). The 2.5 hours a day of pre-school education is interpreted differently by local authorities. While Scottish Executive guidance suggests offering parents some flexibility over the five half-day sessions, enabling them to be compressed into 2.5 days, not all authorities find it possible to do this (Scottish Executive, 2002a).

Other funding for services, again in common with England, comes from the Sure Start funding for children up to three years old, supporting disadvantaged areas and groups, and the National Lottery, through, in particular, the New Opportunities Fund (NOF), which is intended to pump-prime school-age childcare, study support and play opportunities. Unlike England, Scotland has had no specific funding programme to support integrated centres such as Neighbourhood Nurseries or Early Excellence Centres. The development of integrated services at a local level requires the use of a variety of different funding streams, and the planning of services involves estimating the number of parents who may qualify for the Childcare Tax Credit. The head of Early Childhood and Out of School Care at Stirling Council described in an article in 2002 how the establishment of an integrated nursery and out-of-school centre providing for children aged up to 14 years took five separate funding streams: the Pre-School Grant, Childcare Strategy, Sure Start, National Lottery funding and mine regeneration funding (available in areas where coal mining had been discontinued), together with the introduction of a charging policy for children using extended hours provision. She commented: "Each of these funding streams relates to different national government targets and required five separate reports to account for each funding stream" (Kinney, 2002, p 9).

The integration of services was one of the aims of a fund established with Scotland's share of a new Children's Fund announced by the Chancellor of the Exchequer in July 2000. The Changing Children's Services Fund was described as a short-term measure to stimulate better services and better outcomes for children and young people through better-integrated planning and delivery (Hughes et al, 2001). But while a stated goal was developing new and innovative approaches to integrated service delivery, its primary focus was on 'vulnerable young children in deprived communities' and did not address those issues of segregation and fragmentation within early years services that are, in some measure, themselves the product of targeting policies. The need for better-integrated funding is said to remain one of the areas under consideration by the Cabinet Sub-Committee on Children's Services.

Curriculum

Issues of quality and diverse approaches to working with children had fuelled the debate over the separation of education and care through the 1980s and 1990s. We noted earlier that Scotland was included in the new regulatory provisions for daycare services brought in by the 1989 Children Act. These provisions were supplemented by Scottish Office guidance (Scottish Office, 1991). Within its advice on the standards necessary to provide safe and good-quality daycare services, the guidance also described the quality of experience that children should receive in registered daycare. A few years after these standards had come into force, Her Majesty's Inspectors of Schools in Scotland published in 1995 *Performance indicators and self-evaluation for pre-school centres* to encourage all centres offering pre-school education to evaluate their own performance through output-quality standards.

During the same period, increasing government involvement in education led to the introduction of the National Curriculum in England and the less prescriptive 5-14 Curriculum in Scotland. In a climate in which quality was becoming an increasing focus of attention, HM Inspectors of Schools in Scotland published a report on *The education of children under five in Scotland* (1994) followed by the publication of guidelines by Learning and Teaching Scotland. As Wilkinson (2003) has described, the centralist approach involved in government intervention in the curriculum was much debated in Scotland but the *Curriculum framework for children in their pre-school year* (HM Inspectors of Schools in Scotland, 1997) was in general well received largely because of its emphasis on a child-centred approach. The guidance initially covered only children aged four years. However, in 1999 this was extended to three-year-olds, tying in with the extension of part-time pre-school education to three-year-olds.

The 5-14 Curriculum sets out the areas of experience and learning to which the pre-school child should have access. It does not make any specific recommendations for provision; rather, it is a statement of good practice, outlining expectations of those services in receipt of government funding. The framework places pre-school education within a context of lifelong learning, noting that children at three years old bring experiences and knowledge with them. The importance of play is emphasised, both for its own sake and also as a learning opportunity.

Learning and Teaching Scotland, which, since 2000, has advised ministers on the school curriculum for children up to 18 years old, now has responsibility for advising primary schools on the content of the curriculum, and since 1991 (when it was known as the Scottish Consultative Council on the Curriculum) it has published a set of national guidelines. The guidelines cover the ages of

---

Box 4.6: Assessment practices in a Scottish nursery

The assessment system in pre-school services focuses on monitoring progress. A nursery that we visited described assessment in the pre-school years in its information for parents in the following way:

> By careful observation of and listening to your child at play, a confidential ongoing assessment of your child's progress is made throughout the nursery year. It is not to show a record of success or failure but to show the development progress of your child, to show staff areas in which your child may require a little more help by the provision of additional activities or to show where activities require to be extended and made a little more difficult. The record enables staff to match activities to the individual child in ways that have meaning for them, taking account of interests, choices and personal motivation. Confidentiality at all times is ensured.

The attainment of children is not recorded at national level, though some local authorities ask teachers to inform them of progress.

---

five to 14 years (when the curriculum is guided by the Scottish Qualifications Authority through standard grade examinations taken when young people are around 16 years old). The 5-14 Curriculum covers environmental studies (including science, social subjects and technology), information communication technology, personal and social development, health education, language, mathematics, expressive arts, and religious and moral education.

The links between these three curriculum documents (called variously a 'curriculum framework', 'national guidelines' and a 'curriculum for S3 and S4' – third- and fourth-year secondary school pupils, aged 14-16 years) are shown in Table 4.4.

The Scottish Executive and Learning and Teaching Scotland are currently developing a Framework for Care and Learning 0-3. As with all aspects of Scottish education, the 0-3 framework will consist of guidelines, not a set curriculum. The aim of the framework will be to help carers to develop the child's social and interactive skills and to help the child to achieve its full potential, within the context of best possible care and nurturing.

Currently, no curricular guidance exists for leisure and out-of-school services in Scotland. However, out-of-school care services are regulated under the 2001 Regulation of Care (Scotland) Act and as such are subject to national care standards that cover the key areas of dignity, privacy, choice, safety, realising potential and equality and diversity.

Table 4.4: Scottish Curriculum Framework

Curriculum framework 3-5	5-14 Curriculum	Curriculum for S3 and S4 (14-16)
Emotional, personal and social development	Religious and moral education, personal and social development and health	Religious and moral education, personal and social development
Knowledge and understanding of the world	Environmental studies (science, society and technology)	Scientific studies and applications Social and environmental studies
		Technological activities and applications
	Mathematics and applications	Mathematical studies
Communication and language	English language (including a foreign language)	Language and communication
Expressive and aesthetic development	Expressive arts and physical education	Creative and aesthetic activities
Physical development and movement		Physical education
ICT (information and communication technology) (as appropriate in all areas)	ICT (permeating all areas)	ICT (permeating all areas)

Regulation

As we saw earlier, the legislative framework for regulating daycare had become absorbed within English legislation when provisions within the 1989 Children Act replaced earlier Scottish legislation. This anomaly had always made it likely that that this would be an early area for attention. Growing criticism from private and voluntary services over varying standards applied by regulators, and more stringent regulation for these services than existed for nursery schools and classes, made it likely that this would involve centralising the regulatory processes, especially given developments south of the border. In England, the regulatory changes involved integrating the regulation of childcare and schools within a new central regulatory body known as the Office for Standards in Education (Ofsted). In Scotland, the decision was taken to incorporate the regulation of childcare within the regulation of a wider range of services providing care to both children and adults. The regulatory changes were introduced by new legislation in the form of the 2001 Regulation of Care (Scotland) Act, which established the Scottish Commission for the Regulation of Care (Care Commission) and the new Scottish Social Services Council to regulate social work education.

Writing shortly after the 2001 Regulation of Care (Scotland) Act was passed, the Chief Social Work Inspector for Scotland predicted that:

> ... in future the distinctions between many of the staff groups employed in the services regulated by the Commission will break down. For example, as there will be no difference between residential care and nursing home care (both will become care homes) the distinction between social care assistants and nursing care auxiliaries will break down. Similar changes will come for some children's services. (Skinner, 2001, p 7)

However, the opportunities for rationalisation within early years (which now constitutes a substantial proportion of the Commission's work) are more pressing in respect of childcare and education than of care and health, and the new legislation attracted some concern over how it would affect this burgeoning relationship, particularly over inspection (Bloomer, 2001, p 9).

HMIE (Her Majesty's Inspectorate of Education in Scotland) now works alongside the Care Commission to ensure that both the care and the education components of pre-school services are monitored and regulated. HMIE currently inspects nurseries run by local authority education departments. Private daycare and childminders who provide early education are inspected by HMIE with regard to their education provision and by the Care Commission with regard to care. Some pre-school provision will now be required to be inspected by both the Commission and HMIE. However, the legislation stipulates that the Commission will not generally inspect a service in a year that HMIE also carries out an inspection. It is anticipated that the Care Commission and HMIE will work together to ensure that they are both working to the same standards. *The child at the centre* (Scottish Executive, 2000), a self-evaluation guide for all centres providing pre-school education and daycare for children aged from three to five years, forms the basis of HMIE inspections of pre-school education facilities and, since 2003, inspections by the Care Commission. It is based on HMIE performance indicators used in the inspection of centres for what is described as pre-school education purposes, and it was frequently referred to by our interviewees as a 'key document'. The foreword, by the then Minister for Children and Education, referred to taking "education and care as an indivisible whole', as well as regarding 'the experience of the child as being of central importance" (Scottish Executive, 2000, p 3).

Unlike local authorities, which, following the 1989 Children Act, regulated services for children of eight years and under, the Care Commission regulates services for children and young people up to the age of 16. This higher age limit brings more services under regulation, although it still excludes 'own home' care other than the new sitter services (see p 122).

Staff pay and conditions

The services we have been considering continue to be staffed by a variety of professionals and childcare practitioners, including teachers, classroom assistants, nursery nurses, play workers and youth workers. In general, they share only one common characteristic: gender. In common with England, it is a largely female workforce and continues to reflect the separate historical development and continuing fragmented structure of the services (as discussed later).

There is a continuing division between the university-based professional training of pre-school teachers and the industry-based knowledge and competency approach of childcare qualifications such as the SVQ in Early Years Care and Education. Although non-degree courses are available for those who wish to work with children and young people, there is no clear career path for non-teaching staff who wish to become teachers. We found in two of our case studies that new kinds of jobs are beginning to emerge, but some difficulties surrounded some of the new job descriptions. For example, the Schools Department of one of our case study authorities had recently advertised job titles such as 'teacher for children and young people – maths' and 'teacher for children and young people – primary', creating the possibility of a common job title across education provision. However, this had not been viewed favourably by the teachers' trade union. A further development within the same authority whereby pre-school staff were called 'teachers' had stalled due to national-level discussions on the role and pay of nursery nurses.

The deep divide between professionally qualified teachers and the many other vocationally qualified or largely unqualified groups is reflected in levels of pay, conditions of employment and status within the services. This is a divide that many of those we interviewed saw likely to widen in the wake of the agreement with teachers following the McCrone Inquiry (McCrone, 2001) on the future of the teaching, which led to improvements in pay and conditions for teachers. This agreement also regulated the maximum hours to be spent teaching, and also the pension arrangements and professional development of teachers. The subsequent agreement widened the gap between teachers and other workers within services – and, at the same time, by more strictly defining the role of teachers (although envisaging greater flexibility over hours), is likely to have encouraged an expansion of other groups of workers within schools. There are wide differentials in the salaries of teachers (with a starting salary of £16,005 (€22,877) per annum and an upper limit of more than £60,000 (€85,800) per annum) and of non-teaching pre-school staff (recent research shows that supervisors earn less than £15,000 (€21,450) per annum (McCrone, 2001).

Resentment over the gap in pay and conditions between teachers and in particular nursery nurses led to extensive industrial action by nursery nurses in 2003, a dispute that at time of writing remains unresolved.

In general, pay and conditions of childcare workers are significantly better in the local authority sector than in private and voluntary pre-school services. A report published in 2001 by Audit Scotland found:

> Employees in council run centres generally receive higher rates of pay, work fewer hours and have longer paid holidays than those in the private and voluntary sectors. These differences mean that a qualified nursery nurse costs nearly twice as much to employ in the council sector as in the private or voluntary sectors. (Audit Scotland, 2001, p 32)

Training and qualifications

A wide variety of qualifications is available to childcare and education workers (Table 4.5).

Research conducted on training and qualifications by Martin et al (2003) concluded:

> Inter-relationships among existing awards relevant to childcare, early education and playwork are confused and confusing. There is no formal system of accreditation of prior learning in place to allow ease of progression from one award to another. Articulation with higher education is problematic as there is little formal recognition by Higher Education [HE] providers of the value of existing awards. (Martin et al, 2003, p 7)

Fifty per cent of pre-school staff hold the Scottish Qualifications Authority (SQA) Level III. Scottish Executive research into early education and childcare qualifications undertaken in 2000 found that 40% of staff working in Early Education and Childcare did not hold a relevant qualification (Scottish Executive, 2003f). Local authority staff were more likely to hold some form of qualification than those under private or voluntary management: 82% of local authority staff held a qualification compared with 71% of privately managed services and 49% of voluntary managed services (Scottish Executive, 2003f).

There is currently no recognised qualification in out-of-school care, though staff are increasingly required to possess SVQ Level II or III in Playwork. This qualification is obtained by staff currently in employment combining work and study. While there is an SVQ specifically in playwork for over eights, it is not regarded as highly as the early years SVQ by employers. This increases the sense that out of school is on the margins of the provision of children's services; one out-of-school worker commenting that she feels 'completely marginalised'.

The major post-1997 change has been the provision, on a UK-wide basis, of a new qualifications framework through an Early Years National Training Organisation (EYNTO). Occupational standards in the out-of-school sector were the responsibility of another National Training Organisation: SPRITO, the National Training Organisation for Sport, Recreation and Allied Occupations, which has encouraged the development of play qualifications.

NTOs are now being replaced with a smaller number of Sector Skill Councils,

Table 4.5: Childcare and education qualifications

	Qualifications	Length of training
Childminders	None	None
Nanny	SVQ Level III in Early Years Care and Education	12-18 months, carried out while in work
	HNC in Childcare and Education	One year full-time study
Crèche worker	SVQ Level II or III in Playwork	12-18 months, carried out while in work
	HNC in Early Years Care and Education	One year full-time study
Play leader	SVQ Level II or III in Playwork	Work-based qualification taking 12-18 months to complete
	HNC in Early Years Care and Education	One year full-time study
Nursery nurses/nursery assistant/early education and childcare workers	SVQ Level III in Early Years Care and Education	Work-based qualification taking 12-18 months to complete
	HNC in Childcare and Education	
Out-of-school care	None	
Classroom assistants	Professional Development Award	26 weeks part-time including a placement
Special needs assistants	HNC and HND in supporting special learning needs	One year full-time study
Primary teacher	PGCE in primary teaching	One year full-time, following three- to four-year degree programme
	Bachelor of Education	Four years' full-time (study)
Secondary teacher	PGCE in secondary teaching	One year full-time, following three- to four-year degree programme
	Bachelor of Education	Four years' full-time (study)

intended to be larger and to have closer links with employers. This will not include a separate Early Years Sector Skills Council as this sector is said to be too small to justify a separate council. Instead, non-professional early years workers are likely to form part of either a wider Children's Services Sector Skills Council or a wider Social Care Council. In any event, the qualifications framework for non-teachers working in children's services looks set to continue to be separated from the professionally based framework for teachers, the divide being deepened because the former involves a UK framework and the latter is located in Scotland.

Services for children below compulsory school age

The structure of services for children under five-years-old remains diverse and in a number of respects more fragmented. For example, 'sitter services', which were set up to offer informal care to some groups of parents (in particular lone parents and those with disabled children), are now developing in a more formal way through their eligibility for tax credits, which have been extended to cover some care provided in the parent's own home. In addition, the Sure Start programme is stimulating the development of other new kinds of services, including integrated services incorporating childcare, parent support, outreach, play and learning activities (Cunningham-Burley et al, 2002). Childcare Partnerships were envisaged as the means of bringing together this diverse group of stakeholders, 'building on' the existing early years forums; but they are not seen as well placed to serve a particularly strategic role.

As shown in Table 4.1, the pattern and use of services is changing, with a trend towards more use of formal, centre-based care. Total nursery provision increased by 32% from 1997 to 2003, though taking a longer-term view we see that between 1988 and 2003 pre-school nursery provision rose by 151%. Family-centre provision increased by 334% over the period 1997-2003, due at least in part to the funds accessed through Sure Start Scotland. Overall, there is greater use of more formal services for three- and four-year-olds. The number of children accessing playgroups has declined by 56% over the same period, a total drop of 25,822 children, while between 1997 and 2003 the number of children using childminders dropped by 35% and the number using crèche services dropped by 36%. Overall, there was only a modest increase in provision over this period (5.5%, 12,204 children).

There are however, areas of continuity. Local authorities continue to provide the majority of pre-school education services, providing 72% of pre-school education places in 2003 (Table 4.6), significantly higher than the number in England (58%) and reinforcing a view of local authorities as providers of early childhood services. (Local authorities also have a substantial role within general pre-school services – education and daycare combined – with 49% of children who use these services accessing local authority provision.) An HMIE report on standards and quality in the pre-school education provided by different sectors suggests that significant differences exist in the quality of service. Local authority services scored consistently higher across all the areas examined, which included ethos, the curriculum, quality of learning experience, accommodation, resources, staffing, management and quality assurance (HMIE, 2002). The findings raise significant questions about the consistency in quality of the services offered as pre-school education.

The expansion in pre-school education has undoubtedly served to strengthen relationships between schools and pre-school services. However, Scotland has not had any specific funding programmes for integrated services in the pre-school sector, and the New Community School programme has to date led to only limited development of pre-school services and a somewhat greater number

Table 4.6: Number of children in pre-school education by management of centre

	Education (local authority or private schools)		Other non-local authority				
	Local Education Authority (%)	Indepen-dent (%)	Volun-tary sector (%)	Private sector (%)	Other (%)	Total non-education (%)	Total numbers of children
Scotland							
2001[a]	74	–	–	–	–	26	98,937
2002[b]	73	–	11	15	1	27	98,769
2003[b]	72	–	10	17	1	28	105,078
England[c]							
2001	61	5	–	–	–	34	1,156,300
2002	61	5	–	–	–	33	1,142,000
2003	58	5	–	–	–	37	1,195,200

[a] From Summary results of the 2003 pre-school and daycare census (Scottish Executive, published July 2003).

[b] From Provisional results of the 2001 pre-school and daycare census (Scottish Executive, published August 2001).

[c] Provision for children under five years of age in England: January 2003 (Provisional) (DfES, published May 2003).

of pre-school-age services. Nevertheless, the programme is reported to have led to better links between schools and pre-school services, some of which have been included in school 'clusters'. For example, in Glasgow the rolling out of the New Community Schools programme has led to the clustering of nursery, primary and secondary schools into 'learning communities'.

Services for school-age children

Out-of-school provision was described by one respondent as the 'new kid on the block' in children's services – often 'tagged on' to existing responsibilities rather than a core element of the services. Although school-age childcare has a long history in Scotland and started to attract government attention prior to 1997, there were relatively few places. Since then, however, substantial funding has been directed towards a number of separate areas of activity, including out-of-school services, breakfast clubs, and learning and study support services. Funding is fragmented, coming from a variety of different sources, including the Scottish Childcare Strategy with funding via childcare partnerships, NOF, local enterprise companies, community regeneration and health programmes, social inclusion partnerships and the funding of parents through the Childcare Tax Credit, available to cover childcare costs for children up to the age of 15 years, and other help available to lone parents. A Scottish Executive report lists some 15 funding sources for school-age childcare (Scottish Executive, 2003e).

As shown in Table 4.1, the number of places in school-age childcare services has increased significantly, by 14,963 children (108%) over the period 1997-2003, with much of this growth occurring between 2002 and 2003. Most services are provided within schools. *The 2003 pre-school and daycare census* (Scottish Executive, 2003f) found that of the 623 out-of-school care clubs, 330 (53%) were located within school premises. This underestimates the number of schools directly providing out-of-school services as it excludes the large number of 'supported study' or 'homework clubs' that are provided directly by schools on their premises.

The expansion in services has meant that more schools are increasingly in contact of some kind with out-of-school services. Some such services help the schools in an emergency:

> "A couple of times I have actually ended up in the classroom where a couple of teachers have been a bit busy and it's like 'Moira, can you keep an eye on the kids for me for a minute'."

At the same time, some out-of-school staff report being made to feel unwelcome:

> "Out-of-school workers often felt despised by teachers and not made welcome by the head teacher."

> "When I started I wasn't introduced to the staff but got to know them by taking the initiative."

Some report having to help school staff clear up before they can use the premises.

A particular problem for school-age childcare has related to the separate funding streams available for out-of-school learning and out-of-school clubs. (The complexity of funding is known to cause problems, as discussed earlier.)

> "The split means that the out-of-school children, on the same school premises, cannot access 'learning activities' and that while 'care' has to be paid for by parents, learning activities do not."

This problem will be partly addressed through the NOF being asked to prioritise projects that combine childcare with out-of-school learning in a new fund beginning in 2003. A further suggestion made in the Scottish Executive framework report is that of:

> ... using two rooms in a school, with students being able to move freely between them. A study-support room with a programme of structured activities running for an hour or so and a 'chill-out' room in which to socialise, relax and play, open for longer. Staff have playwork and teaching support skills. Outcomes could include improved attainment levels, structured

and informal learning opportunities, and play opportunities appropriate to the children's age. (Scottish Executive, 2003e, p 67)

Out-of-school 'education' provision tends towards study support or homework clubs that, in addition to being free, are staffed by volunteer teachers and are more likely to be open-access. While this educational provision focuses primarily on learning activities, out-of-school care activities often contain within them elements of education; for example, the staff may assist children with their homework. As one interviewee noted:

> "[Homework] is encouraged but parents are asked whether they want the children to do their homework at the club. The children don't have to do it if they don't want to."

The introduction of health-promotion breakfast clubs has introduced a further strand of provision. These provide breakfasts, commonly in areas of multiple deprivation, and are usually free, while other clubs have to charge fees for providing the same services.

Both the framework report and the Coalition Partnership Agreement appear to envisage an increasing role for schools in developing access to out-of-hours activity and facilities for all children (Scottish Executive, 2003a) and accommodating clubs on their premises (Scottish Executive, 2003e). The aspiration to develop access for all children suggests a mainstream service, and the framework document highlights the allocation of £3 million (€4.29 million) to local authorities to allow them to offer ongoing support to services for which start-up funding is due to end. However, the report's emphasis on ways in which services can be helped to become sustainable – including suggestions on how services can be given business consultancy support, and how employers can be involved in subsidising places – highlights their continuing marginality and, in this sense, their separation from schools.

It remains to be seen what will come from implementing the commitment to integrated community schools and the pilot programme exploring alternative structures to the school day, envisaged by the Action Plan from the National Debate on Education. Although there are now closer links between school and school-age childcare services, this has not to date led to any significant rethinking at a national level of the relationship between schools and school-age childcare.

The extent of integration at a local level

Within the Scottish Executive there was a view that the integrative changes at national level had made it easier for local authorities to follow suit. An interviewee described how the Scottish Executive saw itself as influencing reform "by spreading good practice rather than aiming the boot ... and encouraging through funding, such as the Changing Children's Services Fund";

but, while there have been changes at a local authority level, they have varied in nature. As we saw earlier, Scotland undertook the first major initiative to integrate early years services at a local level when Strathclyde Regional Council launched its Pre-Fives Initiative in 1986.

The extent and model of integration varied between our three local authority case studies. In two of them, a number of senior staff had experience of the Strathclyde initiative. This contrasts with what, as we noted earlier, was reported to us as a relative lack of knowledge of the Strathclyde experience within the Scottish Executive. One of our case studies was a successor authority to Strathclyde, with a Director of Education who had been an education officer for pre-fives. The authority had inherited a pre-fives service based within education and in 1998 reorganised its departmental divisions, bringing in play, culture and the arts, out-of-school activities, the toy library and the public library services to the Education Department.

The structure of the second authority is somewhat different. Having developed through the establishment of a children's committee involving a single children's service but with three separate departments (Housing and Social Services, Education Services and Community Services), it subsequently, in 1999, established an integrated children's service bringing together early years education, out-of-school care, compulsory education and social work functions for children. The Children's Services department is one service and is aiming for full integration rather than having one director with strategic responsibility for two separate departments.

A third authority had taken a different approach to integration, retaining the traditional divisions between departments but creating a high level of discussion and joint working. In particular, it has instigated a Joint Committee on Children and Young People and a joint appointment of a Head of Children, Young People and Families with a strategic overview of all services for children and young people. The focus in this authority is on developing new relationships and new ways of thinking, rather than on restructuring and merging. However, strong divisions remain between education and childcare, which are still conceptualised, structured and funded separately.

As we saw earlier, childcare partnerships were intended to provide a vehicle for bringing together the wide range of stakeholders involved in providing or developing early years services, including school-age childcare services. But the partnerships were criticised by voluntary and private providers for being too often chaired by local authorities, while local authorities criticised a lack of willingness by other agencies to take on the work involved. An evaluation carried out in 2000 found that nearly half of all members of the Childcare Partnerships in their study said their role had not been explained to them and expressed concern over the lack of mechanisms available to them to consult with and represent their sector (Blake Stevenson, 2000). The partnerships were based on the principle of involving existing providers; but the evaluation found only a limited involvement on the part of stakeholders such as parents and employers. The partnerships do not appear to have been well constituted to serve an effective strategic role at a local level.

Writing in 2002, the Head of Early Childhood and Out of School Care at Stirling Council noted the complexities of "partnership working within a prescribed model ... exacerbated by the pressures nationally to ensure that local authorities maintained a mixed economy early years sector, as well as ensuring that targets were met in relation to the delivery of places for three- and four-year-olds" (Kinney, 2002, p 8). The sense of confusion that often accompanies rapid change has been compounded for local authorities by the mixed messages they have received:

> The pressure on local authority partnership working increased as separate national strategies were produced. For example, under the early education and quality assurance guidance, local authorities were given greater responsibility for the quality assurance and support to private partners yet the childcare partnership guidance encouraged the authority not to be the dominant partner. The need for greater flexibility in provision was being set out in the Childcare Strategy yet, at the same time guidance on the definition of a part-time nursery education place was expressed as being a 5 x 2.5 hours per week with the effect of limited flexibility. (Kinney, 2002, p 9)

This sense of mixed messages was compounded by the different approach at national level to departmental responsibility and regulation. Departmental responsibilities were brought together within education; regulation was centralised within a social care agency. Moreover, the loss of the regulatory function led in some cases to a loss by local authorities of key staff who over a period of years had become familiar with the issues – just at the time when opportunities were opening up within education for reshaping the relationship between services. New Community Schools, the discussion engendered through the National Debate on Education over the role of schools, and the school-building programme are creating new possibilities and still offer many opportunities.

However, they have not to date succeeded in significantly diminishing the fragmentation within services – and therefore in children's lives – which has for so long bedevilled this area, as seen in the story of a hypothetical child that started this chapter.

Relations with other services

Health

We described earlier the wider policy agenda of the new administration in Scotland following the 1997 UK General Election and the extent to which this intensified after the establishment of the Scottish Parliament, driven by ideas about modernising government, children's rights agendas, and policies on social inclusion and child protection. This has increasingly involved a focus on health.

At a local level the role of health services in both early years and out-of-school provision has been greatly increased during the period of the reforms, fuelled by increasing concern over the health of the Scottish population. The rapid expansion in breakfast clubs was promoted by health department initiatives and funding. Similarly, health services are widening their role; for example, we came across community Healthy Eating Officers who provide information on healthy eating across the area. At a national level, we noted earlier the impact of the Scottish Executive Action team's report *For Scotland's children* and its recommendation that all education, social work and health services for children should be regarded as a single unified service, with the possibility raised of health being given a coordinating role for all services for children under the age of five *before they enter formal education services* (Scottish Executive, 2001a, p 90). We also saw that a proposed draft strategy for the early years published early in 2003 appeared to reflect this. The Scottish Executive is currently taking this agenda further with a review of the child surveillance system in the light of the recommendations of the Hall Report in England (Hall, 2003), which saw Community Health Partnerships as the vehicle for driving forward the recommendation of introducing a standardised approach to child surveillance and child health promotion, linking into early years services, with obvious implications for roles, qualifications, training and pay within the early years workforce.

Culture, leisure and play provision

We found at the local level an increasing emphasis on arts and play associated with both pre-school and school-age services. In one of our local authority case studies, reorganisation brought together not only all relevant early years services (pre-school, school-age childcare and play) but also areas such as arts and culture (including libraries). The profile of the arts field was enhanced by this reorganisation, which also prompted rethinking within educational services of further connections that might be made with arts. One example of this was the use of libraries for NOF-supported study projects. However, the profile of youth workers was generally low. Respondents rarely mentioned youth work specifically; one who did commented that these services had suffered from a lack of investment under previous Conservative governments. These services may now experience an increase in interest, and indeed one Director of Social Work highlighted the importance of these less formal services because young people found them, psychologically speaking, accessible. A further division between youth work and the rest of the field arises from the regulation system. The Commission for the Regulation of Care does not inspect most youth provision, which remains within the local authority system, usually in community learning or similar departments.

Observations

The integration of departmental responsibilities for early childhood education and care services, school and school-age childcare within one division of the restructured Education Department was one of the first measures undertaken by the new Executive following the re-establishment of the Scottish Parliament in 1999. It signalled a determination by the new administration to overcome the split between early years education and childcare services in recognition that the changes initiated at a local authority level – notably by Strathclyde Regional Council in the 1980s – required the support of national policies. Placing both early education and childcare within one division went a step further than the earlier transfer of childcare to the same department in November 1997; "Read my lips", said Sam Galbraith, the then Minister for Children's Issues at a local authorities and early years services conference in 1998, prior to the establishment of a Scottish Parliament, 'integration, integration, integration' (Cohen, 1998).

Departmental reorganisation was one of many changes affecting early years services. The period since 1997 has seen new legislation, new structures, new systems for control and regulation of services and the delivery of training as well as substantial increases in funding.

These changes have also formed part of a wider programme of change affecting policies and services for children. Some of them have stemmed from a growing emphasis on children's rights and have been assisted by a new parliament, which affords greater possibilities for legislative change and participation in the legislative process. More time for effective scrutiny of policies has resulted in the strengthening of children's rights within some legislation, and the establishment of a Children's Commissioner, following an extensive enquiry by parliament.

Some changes have stemmed from the UK-wide 'modernising government' agenda, which was arguably somewhat accelerated in Scotland – at least in terms of departmental restructuring – by the establishment of the Scottish Executive. A public services delivery group, established in the parliament's first term by the McConnell administration, has sought to introduce a client focus to all public services. The integrative agenda for early years has extended outwards and upwards in age, building on a recommendation in 2001 by the Scottish Executive review team (Scottish Executive, 2001a) that all services encompassing education, child welfare, social work, health, leisure and recreation services for children from birth to 18 years should consider themselves as a single unitary system.

Some of the changes reflect the significance that has always been attached in Scotland to education as well as pride in a system that has been seen as "both meritocratic and democratic" (Devine, 1999, p 389). An aspiration to reaffirm its schools as 'world class' has been fuelled by the example of the economic success of the Republic of Ireland, perceived as being in some degree education-led, and this has contributed to a willingness to re-examine the role of schools, seen most noticeably in the New Community Schools initiative and the National Debate on Education. As seen earlier, the possibility of change has also been supported by an extensive new school- and nursery- building and refurbishment programme, offering possibilities for rethinking the use of space within schools and as a shared resource with communities.

Despite these developments, the process of integrating care and education has been affected by a number of wider policies both within and outwith the Scottish nation.

Centralisation and decentralisation in Scottish education and care policy

We have seen how the main strands of early years policy were formulated and put into place at a UK level prior to the establishment of the Scottish Parliament. For example, the Scottish Childcare Strategy differed only in minor respects from the National Childcare Strategy. From the outset, the policy formulated in the National Childcare Strategy significantly constrained the possibility of reformulating the relationship of childcare services with education.

As we saw in Chapter Three, the UK-wide childcare strategy involved some striking continuities with the policies of the preceding Conservative government. This is particularly evident in the market approach taken to the delivery of services for parents in paid employment, combined with subsidies for low-income families provided through the Childcare Tax Credit system. The role of employers in developing childcare has continued to be emphasised. Similarly, the commitment – made at a UK level – to offer all three- and four-year-olds a part-time nursery education place has been delivered on a basis that, while ending the earlier voucher system, continues to support a market approach through offering the possibility of choice between different services and sectors. Justified in terms of 'parental choice' and 'mixed economy of provision', it has underpinned the rolling out of the childcare strategy and perpetuated the concepts of 'pump priming' and support where there is 'market failure'. This UK market agenda sits uncomfortably with the Scottish history of local authority provision.

By contrast, we have seen that some aspects of Scotland's educational policy have been more distinctively its own. In particular, the New Community Schools initiative together with the National Debate on Education offered the possibility of a radical rethinking of the role of schools and those who work in them.

At a local level, the Scottish Executive has taken a less centralised approach to the provision of services than the Westminster Parliament, issuing guidance rather than requirements. On the ground, local authorities retain more control over services. Local authorities have received the funding for the Childcare Partnerships and, unlike England, also for the Sure Start programme. Most childcare partnerships are chaired and managed by the local authority, and have attracted criticism for this. Yet in many ways the most notable characteristic of both Sure Start and the childcare partnerships is that they have in certain respects locked local authorities in as providers within a mixed economy of services, and somewhat constrained the development of integration at a local level. At the moment, the future of childcare partnerships is uncertain. The 2003 draft consultation paper, *An integrated strategy for the early years* (Scottish Executive, 2003b), suggests that their role may be widened but restricted to under-fives.

Targeted and universal services

A further element of the childcare strategy has involved providing integrated support for under threes on a targeted basis. Forming part of the government's social inclusion strategy, the Sure Start Scotland programme has both demonstrated the strength of an inter-agency approach and highlighted tensions between targeted and universal provision and the issues that this can pose for developing non-stigmatised services (Scottish Executive, 2001c).

The focus on providing targeted services has been one of the strongest areas of continuity and seems set to remain so. Sure Start Scotland is aimed at disadvantaged areas, and while every school will now be a community school, the pilot initiative involved targeting of support services – creating some difficulties for schools required to combine universal and targeted elements within their funding agreements (Sammons et al, 2003). Discussions of child surveillance following the Hall Report suggest that health services will also veer towards a targeted approach to service provision (Jackson, 2003, p 6).

Joining up and the wider agenda

'Joining up' has become a national imperative on a much larger scale than might have been imagined in 1999. The joining up of childcare and education has been less evident and indeed seems now to be less of a priority. The advisory group to the Scottish Executive on the implementation of the 1998 Scottish Childcare Strategy no longer meets. A proposed draft integrated strategy for the early years restricts the scope of the strategy to children under five and makes virtually no reference to schools (Scottish Executive, 2003b). Health is currently being considered as the lead agency for all services provided for children under five.

An uncompleted process

At the national level the location of a single division for pre-school childcare and education and school-age childcare within the education department has not yet led to any significant reconceptualising of the relationship between early years and school-age childcare services on the one hand, and the role of schools on the other. The term 'childcare' continues to be used separately from 'early education', as in the title for the Division of Early Education and Childcare within SEED, although a 2003 paper refers to 'care' and 'education' now being seen "as part of the same continuum of services rather than being completely distinct from each other" (Scottish Executive, 2003b).

The association of learning and care has become both implicit and explicit in the recognition by policy makers that pre-school education can now be delivered by a range of services. This is reflected in both the National Care Standard (Scottish Executive, 2002a), and the changes made to the 1956 Schools (Scotland) Code, ending the requirement that public sector nurseries should employ a teacher. Within education, the Inspectorate has become increasingly involved in joint and integrated inspections of care and education; and we received a strong message from the then Minister for Education and Young People over the importance of a 'whole child' approach.

The workforce issues surrounding the education/childcare split – and the issues that beset the Pre-Fives Initiative of Strathclyde Regional Council – largely remain, and are considerable. Developments to improve the training and qualifications of those working in non-education-based services have been, for the most part, undertaken without reference to the education workforce. Similarly, the McCrone Inquiry (2001) on the pay and conditions of teachers, which led to a landmark pay deal for teachers in exchange for greater flexibility in working practices, covered school nursery teachers but made no reference to non-teachers working in pre-school and school-age childcare services and schools. The gap between the education and childcare workforces has widened as a result of the McCrone Inquiry settlement, leading in 2003 to extensive and unprecedented industrial action in Scotland by nursery nurses.

As in England, the regulation of childcare services has been centralised.

Unlike in England, the regulatory function was transferred to the new Scottish Commission for the Regulation of Care set up to regulate all care services. Although an integrated system of registration and inspection has been developed, and national standards for daycare and education (Scottish Executive, 2002a), include the assessment of the development and learning of children (which may be by non-teaching staff), the location of the regulatory function within a social care agency has practically and conceptually reinforced the separation of childcare from education.

Although funding has increased significantly, the separation and multiplicity of funding streams, together with continuing expectations that provision for working parents may require only pump-priming, have continued to constitute formidable barriers to the integration of education and care. The most extensive problem reported at a local level has been that of funding. All three local authorities reported problems with the availability of funding, the difficulties of sustaining new services and the complexity of the funding streams.

While the rhetoric is about integration, funding continues to divide. The framework for the development of out-of-school care (Scottish Executive, 2003e) identified 15 separate funding streams for such care. One interviewee within a childcare partnership spoke also of the concern she and colleagues felt about the focus they are required to give to getting people into employment; "setting up provision for working families to the exclusion of other families".

It is not yet clear what will emerge within Scotland from the distinctive, educational strands of policy. Certainly, Scottish Executive ministers have shown some willingness to distance themselves from discussion in England over the failures of the comprehensive education system. They took advantage of the National Debate on Education to reaffirm their own commitment to the comprehensive system – but also the need for change. The Scottish Executive's response to the debate referred to the need for "radical new thinking about the way we design, build and manage our schools, about the way teachers teach, about the curriculum, and about the interaction between pupils, parents, community and school" (Scottish Executive, 2003e, p 4). The Action Plan includes provision for piloting – with volunteer schools – alternative structures to the school day and enabling teachers to work across primary and secondary schools. The New Community School concept, particularly when reinforced by the new school-building programme, has delivered new relationships and new arrangements – and the potential for new roles. But it has not yet radically reshaped the boundaries between education and care.

Departmental reform has been wider in Scotland than in England or Sweden, but while the focus has moved upwards in age and widened to include services such as health, the split in early childhood services, which was a major factor in prompting reorganisation, remains an obstacle to developing the whole-child, whole-day approach that remained an aspiration for many of our interviewees – including the minister. And we have to conclude that, while Scotland remains locked into the market-led, HM Treasury-determined childcare policies that it shares with the rest of the UK, the impact of some of its educational policies in respect of early childhood services and school-age childcare is likely to be more limited than might otherwise have been the case.

FIVE

Sweden

Farrah's story

Farrah and her family moved to Sweden from Iran in 1998 when she was only two years old. As asylum seekers they arrived with very little money or personal belongings. They now live in a city in the west of Sweden and, although the majority population is Swedish, a fifth of the population in the city were born outside Sweden.

Farrah's father, Adel, works as a mechanic, earning around SEK180,000 (€19,509) per annum, below the national average of SEK191,000 (€20,701) per annum. Around 30% of this salary goes on taxes, but the family receives child benefit at SEK950 (€103) per child per month. Farrah's mother, Zari, like most mothers in Sweden, works part time (and often works overtime), but for relatively long hours: in Zari's case about 30 hours a week at a local grocery shop. Farrah also lives with her younger brother Hamid, who is two years old and attends the local pre-school centre while his mother is working.

Farrah's care and education, from birth to seven years old

Like most young children in Sweden in the late 1990s, Farrah attended the *förskola* (pre-school centre) until she was five years old. She started attending as soon as possible after the family arrived in Sweden back in 1998, as her parents wanted her to settle into her new culture quickly. She spent 35 hours a week in the *förskola*, which like most pre-school centres, was run by the local municipality (*commune*). Her group at the *förskola* had its own rooms, and with 12 children and two adults it had a relaxed and calm atmosphere. Both of the adults were pre-school teachers, trained to degree level in early years childcare and education.

Although there is a national pre-school curriculum, it refers to general principles, such as democracy and openness, and goals, rather than specifying in a detailed way topics to be covered. The goals in the curriculum are broad objectives for teachers to aim for rather than targets that children must reach. Farrah's personal development and learning were not formally assessed, and she learned about the world around her through play and activities. Usually, the group worked with themes, like water or seasons, and constructed activities together around these topics.

The pre-school service was publicly funded with parents paying a means-tested fee, which averaged around a sixth of the total cost. When Farrah's younger brother was born, her parents worried that she would lose her place at the pre-school centre as her mother would be on parental leave and no longer in employment. However, the *commune* introduced a policy to guarantee children the right to continue in pre-schools during parental leave periods, anticipating a new national law that has now extended this right to all children.

At six years old, Farrah went to the local school and attended the non-compulsory pre-school class. Before she moved up to the school, Farrah and her parents were invited to visit the school and meet with the staff. Farrah was at the pre-school class only for the morning and spent the afternoon at home with her mum and little brother. The pre-school class was led by a pre-school teacher with a university degree in education.

Farrah's care and education today, at seven years old

Farrah is currently in her first year of compulsory schooling and attends the local school (*grundskola*) situated a short walk from her home. The school is a whole-day school, which is open from 7am to 5pm, and combines a pre-school class, compulsory schooling and school-age childcare. Her class has 25 pupils. In Farrah's school, children are grouped according to age, but in other schools there are mixed-age groups, including children aged between six or seven and nine. There is a team of adults in the classroom, including two teachers who job-share and a free-time pedagogue (a worker specialising in school-age childcare and more informal education) who works in the classroom at certain times as well as being responsible for school-age childcare provision in the school. There are also often student teachers on practice placement. These student teachers are the first intake of the new teacher training system that brings together the previously separate training of pre-school teachers, school teachers and free-time pedagogues.

Children can arrive from 7am, but the school day itself starts at 8.15am with a quiet time, when most of the class read books of their choice or play quietly. After this, formal teaching begins following the guidance of the National Curriculum for compulsory schooling. The curriculum is based on the principles of democracy and respect for persons. It focuses on encouraging understanding and compassion, openness, the rights and obligations of pupils and their families, and passing on cultural heritage as well as imparting knowledge. In its fundamental values and approach it has much in common with the pre-school curriculum; both offer a broad framework that leaves interpretation and implementation to local authorities, pre-schools and schools.

At 12.30pm the children have lunch, which is provided free of charge. After compulsory school has finished at 1.15pm, Farrah and her friends make their way to the rooms set aside for the leisure-time centre (*fritidshem*) – the school-age childcare service. These are on the school grounds and are laid out specifically for leisure activities, although they are used during the school day as workshops or for one-to-one work with children. This type of school-age childcare service is used by the majority of Swedish children from six years old (when they start school on a voluntary basis) up to and including nine years old: indeed, children of this age are entitled to a place. The degree of integration between classroom and leisure time varies, although as in Farrah's case there is usually some sharing of free-time pedagogues.

Children in school-age childcare are supervised by free-time pedagogues but do not have to do their homework or study. Instead, Farrah spends some of her time in activities planned by the pedagogues and the rest in free play; she often plays outside, for example, climbing trees or tobogganing. Around 40 children attend this centre, along with three staff, all of whom have trained as free-time pedagogues by completing a three-year higher education course. With a salary of SEK15,500 (€1,680) per month, the free-time pedagogues are paid less than the classroom teachers, who currently earn SEK18,500 (€2,005) per month. The service and staff are funded and managed by the *commune*.

Farrah's parents have benefited from the introduction of additional government subsidies for pre-schools and school-age childcare. A family such as Farrah's – with one child at pre-school, the other at school-age childcare – will be charged 3% of their income for the younger child and 1% for the older one, up to a maximum of SEK1,520 (€165) a month.

The head teacher, or *rektor*, is responsible for all aspects of the school, including the free-time centre. He trained as a free-time pedagogue in the 1970s and has been working in the city since the 1980s. *Rektors* are increasingly coming from backgrounds other than school teaching, such as pre-school teachers or free-time pedagogues, though currently they are still in the minority.

Although Farrah is now fluent in Swedish, she is entitled to lessons in Kurdish, her mother language, for four hours a week, as are 12% of the student population in Sweden. Though nationally only 50% of those entitled to this specialist education receive it, the large immigrant population in the city means that the school is able to provide a specialist teacher. Though Farrah likes the teacher and her classmates, she does not like the fact that the mother-tongue lessons are carried out after school, thus eating into her playtime.

In her first year of compulsory schooling, Farrah has been very involved in the school council. She was elected by her class to represent them at the council meetings along with her friend Fredrik. This meeting involves representatives from every class, the *rektor*, some of the class teachers and a representative from the free-time centre. They discuss all sorts of issues at the meetings, including the playground, school-wide activities like open days and, on a regular basis, the school meals. Although the school meals are provided free of charge to the children and the teachers (so long as they sit with the children to eat), and there is always a vegetarian option, the lack of choice and the quality of some of the food is something the children feel quite strongly about. The head teacher has promised to look into the possibility of more options and to raise it with his superior at the municipality.

Farrah's future care and education, from seven to 12 years

Swedish education consists of nine years of compulsory schooling until age 16. Though most children in Sweden move to another school at the end of their fifth or sixth year of compulsory schooling, Farrah is at one of the more recent 'campus' schools that provide education for children from the ages of six to 16 years.

Farrah will be assessed in three ways during compulsory school. Class teachers are obliged to assess each individual pupil's learning and developmental progress and discuss these with the children and their parents. So, at least once a term, the teacher will meet Farrah with her parents to discuss how her learning and social development can best be supported; Farrah will be expected to put forward her own point of view and take some responsibility for her own progress and planning her studies. It is also an opportunity for parents to understand the school better and for teachers to become acquainted with parents' and pupils' experience and opinions and to explain their objectives. Farrah will take national tests in Years 5 and 9, that is, when she is 11 and 15 years old. These tests are nationally standardised and carried out at all schools. The aim is not to give each individual child a test result, but to give the teachers support in their assessments and future grading of the children. Formal grades are not given until the last two years of compulsory school, Years 8 and 9. Teachers conduct the grading internally, awarding grades according to pupils' knowledge and achievements in Swedish, mathematics and English. This is part of the new goal- and knowledge-related system that ensures that almost every pupil is given a leaving certificate. Since only 1% of pupils fail to receive a final grade, Farrah's parents are not too concerned. They are sure that she will go on to the local *gymnasium* (or upper school for young people aged 16 to 19 years) where she will finish her schooling.

Chapter Two indicated some of Sweden's distinctive political, social and demographic features and ways in which it resembles and differs from England and Scotland. We discussed Sweden's strong attachment to the values of equality and democracy, reflected in characteristics such as low levels of child poverty and a more equal distribution of income than in England and Scotland. Sweden is a relatively wealthy society, though no more so than England and Scotland overall; it is also a world leader in the development and use of information technology (Moss and Petrie, 2002). We saw that there are high levels of employment, including among women and mothers, and a typically Nordic welfare regime that allows for the provision of universal welfare services, including childcare. High taxes produce high benefits, including impressive policies on leave, public provisions for children and low levels of child poverty. It is important to remember, also, that Sweden has a growing minority ethnic population.

Sweden is a very large country in terms of its total area, but is somewhat sparsely populated. The 289 *communes* are very diverse, ranging from large industrial urban areas to small fishing towns and vast forested areas that reach into the Arctic Circle. The *communes* can be very small by British standards; for example, one of those we visited consisted of 14,000 inhabitants, while there are also the larger cities with 100,000 inhabitants and more. Swedish decentralisation policy leaves much responsibility at this level.

Of special relevance to our study of the integration of services is the long-standing, often vigorous debate on the place of children in Swedish society and on the meaning of childhood. This is a debate that is framed in prevailing understandings of equality and democracy.

Terms

At the outset of this chapter, we must say something about the specialist terms that are used in Sweden. Words that seem to translate neatly from one language to another do not necessarily do so in fact, and for others there are no exact equivalents. Each society has its own institutions that never exactly match those of other societies; even institutions seemingly as commonplace as schools have different histories and different organisational forms, and have different meanings for those who use them and work in them. So, as readers and writers, we have to be especially careful in the use of terms and not impose our own meanings, inappropriately, upon the provision to be found elsewhere, difficult though this may be. For the Swedish case study, specialist terms concerning school, childcare and education will be used as defined below – and this glossary will also provide an initial background to services that, we hope, will be of use in the rest of the chapter.

Pre-schools (*förskola*) are centres for children aged from one to six years prior to the reforms described in the case study, and for children aged from one to five years today. The centres provide integrated childcare and early education, full-time. From 2004, children aged four and five years have the right to free pre-school activities (three hours a day).

Pre-school classes (*förskoleklass*) are for children aged six years. Before the reforms described here, these children were in pre-schools. Now they are in these classes in the *grundskola* (to be discussed later). These classes are attended on a voluntary basis and precede the first of nine years of compulsory schooling.

Children who attend the pre-school class also often attend the free-time services based in the same school (to be discussed later).

Free-time services (*fritidshem – fritids* for short) is used to describe school-age childcare provision – the 'free-time home' as distinguished from other free-time (leisure) activities such as sports or music facilities that are separate from the school and do not offer a care service but are also described as *fritids*.

Family daycare (*familjedaghem*) in Sweden mainly includes childminders who are employed by the *commune*.

Compulsory school (*grundskola*) is the compulsory or basic school, compulsory for all children aged from seven to 16 years. Mostly this stage of schooling is split into two phases with grades 1 to 5 or 1 to 6 forming one phase and grade 6/7 to 9 the second phase. A less usual, but increasingly common, pattern is for grades 1 to 9 plus the pre-school class to be organised on the same site with the same head teacher.

Attendance at upper secondary school (*gymnasie skola*) is not compulsory, but almost all (95%) young people aged 16 to 19 attend. The upper secondary school provides three-year academic and vocational courses. Students must pass examinations in Swedish, English and mathematics, in their compulsory schools, in order to obtain a place. There are further requirements for those wishing to study the more academic subjects.

A school principal (*rektor*) is the head of a compulsory school with its associated pre-school class, free-time care services and in some cases one or more local pre-school centres and some family daycarers. A school principal may have, initially, a teaching qualification for school or pre-school or a qualification as a free-time pedagogue. The head of an upper secondary school (*gymnasium*) is also titled *rektor*.

A free-time pedagogue (*fritidspedagog*) works in free-time care services and supports children's education (in the widest sense of the word) and well-being. He or she also works alongside the compulsory school teacher and the pre-school class teacher during the school day. With the reforms of teacher education, to be described later, a separate education for the pedagogue no longer exists, and the profession is to be merged with that of teacher.

A pre-school teacher (*förskollärare*) works in pre-school and in pre-school classes and, like the free-time pedagogue, until the reforms had a separate education from that of the teacher.

Childcare assistants (*barnskötare*) work in pre-schools and other settings. Training for this occupation used to be provided by the upper secondary school, but this is no longer available and the occupation is declining.

The term 'pedagogy' will be used, as in Sweden, to relate to education in its broadest sense, involving the whole child – social, physical, emotional and intellectual – rather than in the narrower sense in which it is often used in the English language, when it is confined to the sphere of more formal learning and education.

Commune will be used to translate *commune,* the local authority, to which much power is devolved in Sweden.

Background to reform: services and change prior to 1996

Until 1996, early years and school-age childcare services were the responsibility of the Ministry of Social Affairs and the National Board of Health and Social Welfare, while the Ministry of Education and the National Agency for Education (*Skolverket*) were responsible for compulsory schooling.

All of these services were, and continue to be, publicly funded, with some contribution from parents towards childcare services, and for the most part provided by the public sector. There is also publicly funded provision outside the public sector. The 'free-school' system established during the 1990s allows parents, staff, non-profit organisations (and even profit-making companies in some circumstances) to start and run pre-schools, free-time care services, compulsory schools and upper secondary schools. These, if they meet the standards required, may obtain public funding similar to that obtained in the public sector and offer staff the same pay and conditions.

In Sweden, state schooling was in place by 1842, eventually reaching its current provision for children between the ages of seven and 16 years, and addressing the formal educational needs of the child. The history of Swedish early childhood services also has its roots in the 19th century and manifests two main concerns: the amelioration of the health and well-being of poorer children, often addressed by charitable organisations and, later, *folkbarnträdgärd*, public kindergartens which provided for children from all social classes and integrated concerns for children's general well-being, learning and development.

Free-time centres were available, in some localities, from the late 19th century. Responsibility for these was assumed by the Ministry for Social Welfare in 1933. Most of the forerunners to the modern *fritidshem* were the result of private initiatives, in fact, as social welfare services. In the period following the Second World War, it was usually pre-school teachers who worked in free-time centres: an indication of the early relationship between early childhood and school-age childcare services. The first training specifically for what became known as free-time pedagogues was introduced only in 1965 and was conducted in the upper secondary schools, mainly for 16- to 19-year-olds, but also in adult education. During the 1970s, education for free-time pedagogy was taken into the universities and was usually jointly organised with education for pre-school teachers.

Sweden's high level of childcare provision – for both pre-school and school-age children – began to build up from the early 1970s. This was for two interconnected reasons: to meet the needs of working parents and to promote gender equality by enabling women to join the workforce. From as early as 1975, an obligation was placed on *communes* to provide early childhood and school-age childcare services for children from one to 12 years where parents were employed or studying, and for children with additional needs – for example, disabled children. This obligation was strengthened and extended by subsequent legislation. Services – pre-schools, family daycare and free-time care services – were publicly funded, but with parents paying fees. Among these different forms of provision, pre-schools and free-time care services have predominated, and family daycarers have played a lesser part. From the mid-1970s, levels and take-up of childcare provision expanded rapidly. This was associated with high male and female employment, until this was affected somewhat by the recession of the early 1990s, to which we return later.

Three important elements of the context in which the reforms occurred need to be raised before we proceed to the immediate history and processes of reform: the influence of the United Nations (UN) Convention on the Rights of the Child, the decentralisation of decision making from central to local government and the long-standing discussion on pedagogy and learning.

The UN Convention

Box 5.1: Measures accompanying Sweden's ratification of the UN Convention on the Rights of the Child

- A decision was made that implementing the Convention was to be an active policy that permeates all ministries, and is not confined merely to ministries with immediate responsibilities to provide for children.
- The Convention was to be incorporated into training and in-service training of professionals and *commune* employees.
- All government decisions should be subject to child impact analyses so as to discover how any policy affected children.
- The role of the Children's Ombudsman, already in existence, should be reviewed and strengthened.
- The child's perspective should be included in the terms of reference of commissions of enquiry and similar bodies.
- The influence and participation of children and young people should be developed in social and traffic planning.
- Statistics about children should be further developed.

Sweden has taken a strong position on the UN Convention on the Rights of the Child, and one of our informants described it as a 'hot topic', that is, one that carried weight and had been in the forefront of developing policy.

The measures accompanying Sweden's ratification of the Convention must be seen within a social context that places a strong explicit value on democracy. For example, the curriculum for the compulsory school begins:

> Democracy forms the basis of the national school system. The 1985 Education Act (p 1100) stipulates that all school activity should be carried out in accordance with fundamental democratic values and that each and everyone working in the school should encourage respect for the intrinsic value of each person as well as for the environment we all share. (Swedish Ministry of Education and Science, 1994, p 4)

As one of our informants, an influential academic, said:

> "We want the children to be critical and to question the authority of the grown-ups. The curriculum states just that. Democratic value says that we want people to make their voices heard and to affect their lives and be part of the democratic process. That is a general value in Swedish society. We don't want children to grow up and just wait for the authorities to tell them what is allowed. We want them to question and make their own decisions."

Signs of this approach are also apparent in the plan of one of the pre-schools that we visited (see Box 5.2).

The plan is an official document in which the pre-school has to address how it will, among other duties, foster democracy, children's influence and responsibility. In the plan shown here the children are seen as capable of participating in pedagogical planning, having some responsibility for how and what they learn. This connects with how the school, and Swedish society in general, constructs the child.

Decentralisation

Placing a high value on social agency is to be found in many aspects of Swedish society. One sign that the adult population in Sweden values democratic participation is the high turn-out at local elections. In one of the local authorities we studied, we were told that 85% of the population voted in the last election (although this must be compared with the 40% who voted in the European Union election). The municipal, national and regional elections are all held on

---

Box 5.2: Pre-school plan: the fostering of democracy, children's influence and responsibility

At [pre-school] we will lay the foundation for the children's understanding of democracy. The children's social development requires them to take responsibility according to their ability.

By the fostering of democracy we mean that the children acquire an increased influence and responsibility as their abilities grow.

By responsibility we mean everything, from the youngest child clearing their plate, cutlery and cup and putting them on the trolley...

By influence we mean everything from the youngest child choosing which song to sing in assembly to the elder children being able to participate in pedagogical planning.

the same day and voters are not required to hold Swedish citizenship in order to be able to vote in municipal elections.

An interpretation of democracy that is current in Sweden is that decision making should be made at the most appropriate level. We have already noted, in Chapter Two, one example of this: the recent strong process of decentralisation from central government to *communes*, which exercise key responsibilities for the organisation and delivery of services. Central government provides broad and general policy frameworks, which *communes* then have wide discretion in interpreting and implementing. Because of the strong tradition of decentralisation and professional autonomy, reforms cannot be prescribed and decreed: much depends on negotiation, persuasion, acceptance of different perspectives and being able to carry local people – professionals and staff – along if there are any significant changes in practice and organisation.

Education has been part of this process of decentralisation. In 1991 the *communes* became responsible for education and received large block grants from central government for the provision of schools. But because this grant was not increased to meet the extra costs involved in rising school rolls and an increase in teachers' salaries, the resulting funding shortfall was partly responsible for decisions to carry out the local reorganisation and integration of services to be described later. Today, each *commune* is statutorily obliged to produce an education plan, within the national framework for education, that takes into account national goals and curricula (to be discussed later). However, the *commune* is free to adapt these plans in accordance with local conditions and needs. Thus, the way schools should be organised is not prescribed: local politicians under the guidance of the Director of Education take these decisions.

Decentralisation also extends to individual institutions. Many schools are now governed by local boards with parents in the majority. This measure is promoted because '"the whole of society rests ultimately on man's participation in democracy" (SOU, 1995, p 103). While ultimate responsibility still rests with local politicians, the local boards have the right to decide upon the distribution of school hours and holidays and to be responsible for pupils being offered an all-round selection of subjects to choose from. Other tasks, which are the responsibility of the headmaster but may be transmitted to a local board, include decisions on: open-air activities, the school's work plan, the shaping of the work environment, staff development, development of cooperation between school and family, and anti-bullying policy. While some research studies show positive evaluations of the parental boards (for example, Ritchey, 1998), other work suggests that the boards may develop in different ways. For example, they may take responsibility for very practical aspects of school life, such as local traffic control and school meals, or at the opposite extreme enter the pedagogic domain and consider educational and quality questions (Kristoffersson, 1998).

Informants at local level seemed to welcome the ability to make their own decisions. At the same time, some of them pointed to results of decentralisation that were less palatable. For example, some were of the opinion that decentralisation threatened the equality of children's education across Sweden. Before decentralisation, central state control had meant that the budget for children in all *communes* was comparable. The ability of *communes* to control budgets had made for greater differences in the funding of local education departments. This arose because local political priorities could result in some education departments being disadvantaged in some areas and privileged elsewhere. However, *Skolverket* (the National Agency for Education), which exercises some central control over local education through an inspection system, was seen as a check against disparities becoming too great (this topic is discussed later). Another problem arising from decentralisation and mentioned by schoolteachers was the lack of uniformity in marking tests for entrance to upper secondary school. This could lead to inequalities between schools and between *communes*, a situation that needed to be addressed centrally. Problems associated with decentralisation were expressed strongly by one local politician. We quote below an example of a counterview to what seemed to be the more general appreciation of the move to decentralisation.

> Municipal reform has been important. The school has become less of an issue for the state and is now more the business of the *commune*. One problem has been teachers' pay, which is now decided at the level of the *commune*. Because of the shortage of teachers, very young teachers in scarce subject areas, like mathematics, are now being paid more than experienced teachers. This causes problems.... The system cannot survive; we must go back to state regulation – this is the greatest challenge ahead of us. We don't like the state to make decisions but we are one of 289 *communes*. We cannot be effective unless we are regulated and standardised at national level.

Pedagogy and lifelong learning

Providing childcare for the children of working parents has been a powerful theme in Swedish policy. But it would be misleading to paint a picture in which the function of services, prior to integration, was seen predominantly in terms of childcare. Ongoing discussions of the meaning of the child and childhood, and of pedagogy and of learning, exerted a potent influence on policy. Alongside the development of public provision for children as a means of facilitating parental employment and thus increasing the workforce, Sweden has long placed an emphasis on pedagogy. The term 'pedagogy' is used in Sweden, as in much of Europe, to denote the education of children in the broadest sense of the word. Indeed, from their earliest days, pedagogic concerns have always informed pre-schools and school-age care services.

Pedagogy as used in Sweden is a far from simple, uncontested concept, and different Swedish interviewees emphasised different aspects of it. One, for example, quoted the new pre-school curriculum, which speaks of a 'pedagogical approach where care, nurturing and learning together form a coherent approach', and said that this echoed the thinking of the 1968 Commission (cited later in this chapter). For this informant, the caring component of pedagogy should not be undervalued. She acknowledged that some may see the term 'care' as referring narrowly to the direct physical care of dependents and/or to the field of targeted welfare services. But she found that the problem with these limited meanings contributed to an image of the child as predominantly poor or needy. Our informant held that 'care' was a far richer and more extensive term, relating to human existence as a whole. She said that "to care for humans is what we have to do" and that caring was an essential component of pedagogy. She was in favour of seeing work with children as pedagogy rather than as teaching, because pedagogy introduced a dimension that was not present in teaching. Care, she believed, was more related to an ethical relationship with our world, to being human beings in the world. She thought that in order to reform education it was necessary to start with such ethical considerations rather than epistemological considerations based on knowledge and the realm of teaching. For her, starting from an ethical base implied seeing work with children primarily in terms of relationships, working with them as 'other' and welcoming the differences between them and oneself as worker and adult.

A different emphasis was provided by those informants who spoke of pedagogy in terms of learning, and in some cases observed that applying 'learning' to settings outside the formal classroom was a somewhat recent development in Sweden. (They may not have denied that pedagogy had a care component, but in interview this was not where their main interest lay.) A researcher working in the field of teacher education said that when he had begun his career learning was not a current concept in early childhood education. At that time, learning was not seen as an appropriate aim for the pre-school, and found a place only when children entered the compulsory school system. In contrast, play was seen as the main and proper activity for pre-school children, that is, for children up to the age of seven.

Two particularly important state committees were cited by informants as part of the essential pedagogic background to the reforms: the 1968 Commission on Childcare (*Betänkande avgivet av 1968 års Barnstuge-Utredning*) and the 1969 Commission on the Work of Schools (*SIA-utredningen, the Internal Work of Schools*). The commissions continued their work until 1974. Although focused on different areas – childcare and schools – both adopted a similar holistic approach to the child. Many of their ideas can be traced back to the early part of the century or before: for example, from notions of an 'active pedagogy' in the early 20th century to 'laboratory pedagogy' and 'dialogue pedagogy' in the 1960s and 1970s, all of which, in different ways, presented an image of children as participants in their own education, exploring, active and experimenting. Such ideas are in opposition to another, more subject-focused educational tradition, in which academic disciplines have an essential authority of their own, with knowledge and skills being the domain of experts who impart them to children.

The second report went beyond its remit for the school. It emphasised that it was necessary to look at the whole ecology of childhood and childhood services. It also questioned the prevailing methods to be found in schools and spoke of the need for a more interesting school life for children, and a change in pedagogical methods so that there would be less 'lecturing children' and a more questioning approach. This indicates one of the major issues expressed about the reforms we are about to describe: the tension between subject and skills learning as an end in itself – more typical of the traditional school – and the more humane values that had been of importance in Swedish pre-school and school-age childcare services.

A Swedish informant set out in more detail the significance of the Commission on Childcare:

> "The 'revolution' in pedagogic thinking came with the report on pre-schools in 1972, when the 1968 Commission on Childcare formulated a new theoretical approach to learning in pre-school and, in 1974, also in school-age childcare. This approach was based on the theories of Jean Piaget, Erik Homburger Erikson and George Herbert Mead and influenced by the writings of Paulo Freire, the 'Russian psychologists' (Vygotsky, Luria and Leontjev), Jerome Bruner, and others. This approach put the emphasis on dialogue and mutual exchange of experiences, play, exploratory and laboratory learning and on starting from the interests, views and pre-existing understandings of the children. This approach was then followed up and elaborated by research, developmental work and accompanying texts. For example, in 1975 the National Board of Health and Welfare published a series of books under the joint heading Working Plan for Pre-schools, with titles like *We learn from each other* and *We explore and discover*. The books were meant to explain the 'new approach' to pre-school teachers."

In 1981, a policy document, *The pedagogical work of pre-schools – goals and directions* (*Förskolans pedagogiska verksamhet – mål och inriktning*), was published by the National Board of Health and Welfare. It clearly states that pre-schools have educational aims and meanings and sums up the main educational work of the pre-school (based on ideas from the 1968 Commission on Childcare). This document was the first step in a new approach to curriculum work, moving away from detailed prescriptions directed at teachers and instead stating the main goals, ideas and directions for the *communes* to elaborate in their pre-schools. This was also the starting point for the curriculum work during the 1980s that resulted in Educational Programme for Pre-school in 1987 and Educational Programme for School-Age Childcare in 1988 (Flising, 2003).

Related to this view of the pre-school and free-time services as sites for education are the rather more recent notions of 'lifelong learning'. In Britain we are, perhaps, more used to this phrase as applied to learning after the end of compulsory schooling and higher/further education. In this sense it is often used to refer to regular retraining of the workforce as a means of promoting labour market mobility and competitiveness. In Sweden, too, lifelong learning has been promoted as a means of enabling Sweden to compete as a knowledge-based society within the global economy. But learning, it is emphasised, is an important domain for all human beings. This is a viewpoint used to justify the introduction of children into educational establishments from at least the age of one year, and certainly before the start of compulsory schooling. 'I think it's a good thing that we see life as an integrated learning period', said one of our informants, who thought that it would be misleading to limit understandings and public policy towards learning to the ages of six to 16 and obligatory schooling. In this conversation he was thinking especially about the earliest provision for learning rather than learning in later life. Aspirations for a population for which lifelong learning is desirable were part of the context that allowed the pre-school to be brought under the auspices of education. The education plan of one of the *communes* we studied stated that the pre-school and the compulsory school must become 'meeting places for lifelong learning', and went on:

> In pre-school/school learning will be developed as an unbroken process for each child/pupil. It is the responsibility of pre-school/school to develop and preserve children's interest and enthusiasm for lifelong learning as well as their curiosity. Pupils will be encouraged to start from their own interest and participate in taking responsibility for their own learning. This assumes that the learning processes are planned and carried out in close collaboration between personnel, pupils and parents.

Nevertheless, learning is not the only basis for the pre-school pedagogy. The first sentence of the section that addresses development and learning states:

> The pre-school should be characterised by a pedagogical approach in which care, nurturing and learning together form a coherent whole.

Institutions affected by the reforms

Three distinct institutions, with their own staff, cultures and discourses, were to be radically affected by the reforms of the 1990s: pre-schools, the free-time services (school-age childcare), and the schools themselves. The 1990s were to see increasing integration of all of these services, not only at the administrative level but also in relation to organisation, curricula, funding and staffing. Nevertheless, their separation had come under scrutiny long before any move was made to integrate them as a matter of national policy. By the late 1980s, with increasing numbers of children attending pre-schools and free-time services, their relationships with compulsory schooling were being given much consideration.

Many influential documents, published in the decades immediately preceding the reforms, scrutinised the concepts that underlay public provision for children. These documents were often the work of commissions, bodies of informed people who met and debated over several years before publishing their conclusions. The tradition of public commissions can be seen as part of the democratic process that is so highly valued in Sweden (as discussed earlier). Thinking about and discussing issues fundamental to public policy seems to be an accepted part of Swedish culture. For example, there had long been a debate (since at least the 1940s) on the best age for children to start school and a long-standing discussion, from at least the early 1970s, as to whether to integrate pre-schools into the school system.

Some of the discussion had been in terms of whether pre-school services were essentially a matter of social welfare or of early childhood education. Many pre-school organisations and experts in the field had been against taking these services into education for fear of losing their distinctive identity and because of the perceived threat that the values and methods of the school would predominate. However, others wanted the influence and understandings of pre-schools and free-time services to be brought to bear on schools, which were sometimes characterised as too formal in their approach to children and learning. It was less feasible for them to be influential from a position outside the education system.

These debates were not merely hypothetical but based on concrete and developing experience in the *communes*. Decentralisation made this 'bottom-up' approach to policy development increasingly possible in Sweden, and much of the recent history of reform has been of local developments later taken up at national level. For example, different Swedish *communes* had introduced 'integrated schools' and 'whole day schools' that offered various models of service provision. A school might provide early childhood services, school-age childcare and schooling for children aged from one to 12 years. In these cases, it was possible for children to be located in one establishment throughout their pre-teen years. Other *communes*, which did not necessarily offer pre-school provision, were basing the free-time service in the school. Such experiments could offer children and parents continuity of service over the course of the school day in that children did not have to travel backwards and forwards between the school and the free-time service.

These sorts of provision were often based on teamwork between the different professionals involved: not merely between distinct services within the same setting but between different staff working together with the children, sometimes in small groups, sometimes with whole classes or mixed-age groups, during the formal school day. The desirability of teamwork had emerged as a pedagogic theme from the 1970s (SOU, 1974: 53). A strong argument for integration, based on experience with integrated schools, was the spread of the pedagogic principles that had been developed in pre-schools and free-time services, which might then (from some points of view) improve the educational thinking and working methods of the compulsory school.

Discussion also arose at this time over the cost-effectiveness of school-age childcare, then mostly provided in the *fritidshem*, literally, the 'free-time home', which came under the auspices of welfare and was usually based outside the school and quite independent of it. The free-time care services were recognised as being of very high quality, with highly trained staff employed on a full-time basis. Yet the expensive *fritidshem* stood empty during the school day. In 1985, a commission had failed to suggest any changes to the current system and had in fact recommended that these centres should be further expanded. The government saw this recommendation as unhelpful and therefore did not act on the report's conclusions. In 1989, Göran Persson, then Minister for Schools, appointed a second commission whose terms of reference were to stimulate a more a coordinated approach between schools and the *fritidshem* and to bring the two systems together. Unusually, the commission was given a budget to offer funding for the *communes* to develop initiatives that would address this reform. Targeted funding is one of the ways in which the state can maintain influence in a decentralised system.

These measures, together with the recession of the early 1990s, led to more free-time services being located within schools rather than in more expensive separate provision. This meant that free-time services became more oriented towards the school and less to the pre-school – although in national terms pre-schools and free-time services both still came under Welfare.

Quite rapidly, the encompassing role of the school began to build up. It was also apparent in the integration of the pre-school class (non-compulsory but attended by the majority of children aged six years) into the school in many *communes* (for example, in Skurup and Skövde, from 1991). This was often for economic reasons, but there was also a pedagogic discussion as to the age at which compulsory schooling should begin, whether at six or seven years. Bringing six-year-olds into the pre-school class within the school was often considered in the context of this debate. Some parties urged the benefit of what could be seen as an extra year of schooling for children attending the pre-school class at six; others believed that the formal setting of the school was not suitable for such young children. By the late 1980s, the Ministry of Education wanted provision for six-year-olds, which then came under the auspices of the Ministry of Social Affairs, to be moved to Education. One of our interviewees remarked that the Ministry of Social Affairs had been very reluctant to agree to this, valuing as it did its own pedagogic tradition, while the Ministry of Education was keen to take over responsibility for six-year-olds. The main trades union involved (*Lärarförbundet*) favoured these pre-school children coming within the compulsory school system, as did the Association for Swedish Local Authorities (*Svenska Kommunförbundet*). By the time national responsibility for pre-schools was transferred to education, many of the *communes* had already brought six-year-olds into school-based pre-school classes.

One of the *communes* we studied, where the pre-school class had been brought quite early into the school, saw itself as leading the way in this. By the mid-1990s nearly all of its six-year-olds were in school, compared with 7% in the rest of country. We were told that the integration had started from the needs of the children. The *commune* had at one time called schools where there was an integrated pre-school class 'children's schools', to emphasise that the school was for the child rather than the child for the school. Integrating the pre-school class into the school was more than, and different from, merely starting school at the age of six. The *commune* wanted to build on what they saw as the needs of the children: physical exercise, tranquility, stimulation and creative learning. Meeting these needs was a matter for teachers, free-time pedagogues and pre-school teachers working together towards common goals, integrating the child's day, combining different activities and working thematically. The pedagogic ideal expressed by an informant working in this *commune's* education department was similar to that we met in other settings. She said that children in the pre-school class should be responsible for their own work and for planning it, and should have a choice about the level at which they want to work. The intention was to have a process-oriented view of knowledge so that staff had to ask what kind of knowledge children needed in a world in which today's knowledge is 'perishable goods'.

At a practical level, informants said that situating the pre-school in the school meant that children could more gradually get used to a bigger setting with more and older children, and a different ethos. However, a more school-based rationale was also put forward by some who said that the pre-school class gave children 10 years in school and therefore more time to work towards the goals of the curriculum.

Financial considerations

Alongside pedagogical reasons for change, there were also economic grounds for integrating services. The economic rationale became more pressing with the recession of the early 1990s and carried some weight with the government of those years. In the English summary of her PhD thesis, Birgitta Lidholt observes:

> In the public sector, childcare is one of the areas where the most stringent economic measures have been taken. This means that, in the 90s, group size in many pre-schools increased from 15–16 children to 20–22 children while at the same time staff to child ratio was reduced.... In the early 90s there were vigorous protests in the media against the cutbacks. Staff and parents in some pre-schools were very worried and spoke of crisis and chaos. In a series of articles, 'Pre-school Crisis', published in the Swedish newspaper *Expressen* of 16, 17 and 18 February 1994, the staff of a daycare centre in Biskopsgården, a suburb of Gothenburg, were given the opportunity to express their opinion. Headlines such as 'Goodnight daycare centre. And good morning parking lot for children' – 'Pedagogy? There is no time for that!' shows to some extent how the staff could view the prevailing conditions. (Lidholt, 1999)

Lidholt notes that, because of pressures on the *communes* to balance their budgets, costs per child in pre-school centres decreased by 20-25% in the period 1991-96. She also remarks that costs continue to fall. The main way to save money is to reduce staffing numbers. *Skolverket* has documented a 25% increase in the number of children per worker in pre-schools between 1990 and 1999 and a doubling in free-time services over the same period.

Merging of trade unions

Further evidence of the move towards the integration of services, prior to national legislation, is provided by the amalgamation of trade unions. In 1991 the unions for teachers, pre-school teachers and free-time pedagogues merged as the *Lärarförbundet*. The membership of the new union did not include family daycarers. The merger was reached after about 20 years of discussion between the different groups. A major motivation behind it was to create a strong union for negotiating with the *communes* – responsible since decentralisation for all services – over salaries, working conditions and the education and training required for staff.

However, although teachers and other pedagogical staff might belong to the same union, this did not mean that they enjoyed absolute parity of status. In general terms, the younger the children with whom these professionals worked, and the more general and holistic their work, the lower their status and the less favourable their pay and conditions of employment, such as working hours and yearly timetable. Conversely, those working with older children and young people, and those teaching specialist academic subjects, enjoyed higher pay and better working conditions (as discussed later).

Something of these divisions is evident from the fact that most teachers at upper secondary level and many teachers in compulsory secondary schools were, and continue to be, in a separate union, *Lärarnas Riksförbund*.

Summary: the Swedish system prior to reform

In 1989, Göran Persson, as Minister for Schools, impressed by the *communes'* experiments with integrated services, proposed the creation of a joint national curriculum for all children from one to 16 years of age and to increase cooperation between, or the integration of, pre-schools, schools and free-time services. In 1991, a new Conservative government intervened and for four years there was little further action at national level. This was to change with the election of a Social Democrat government in 1995 and the rapid consolidation of integrated services and staffing within the education system. The reforms' background, which we have described, presents a complex picture of pragmatic, political, social, cultural, financial and pedagogic factors. To sum up, the key features of the Swedish system prior to the 1996-98 reform included the following:

• high levels of publicly funded and publicly provided childcare, free-time care services and early education for children whose parents were employed or studying (that is, the vast majority), together with a statutory entitlement

to parental leave. This meant that most children between the ages of one and 10 years attended pre-school and free-time care services;
- a field that was and is strongly influenced by a welfare regime that emphasises the universal rights of social citizenship, comprehensive risk cover, generous benefits and egalitarianism;
- the decentralisation of decisions about the organisation of local services to the *communes*, many of which recognised the financial, practical and pedagogical benefits of integrating services, and had experimented with different forms of integration. So, in the period shortly before national integration, there was much local integration and some state funding in support of this;
- a workforce across teaching, pre-school and free-time care services that was often working in the same settings and often belonged to the same union, but with different pedagogical cultures (or discourses) and status differentiation manifest in different levels of pay, different lengths of training and education, different time schedules (both weekly and over the year) and other working conditions;
- a long-standing professional and academic debate on the place of children in Swedish society and on broad pedagogical issues, promoted and sustained by the reports of influential commissions; and
- the Swedish system of welfare, based on full labour-market participation with equal opportunities for both mothers and fathers. Recession and a rise in unemployment in the early 1990s stretched national and *commune* budgets and led to cuts and some perceived fall in standards in children's services.

The process of reform

From welfare to education

The local integration of responsibility for pre-schools and free-time services within education was widespread by the time national responsibility was integrated within the Ministry of Education and Science. In 1995, with the Social Democrats back in government and with Göran Persson as Prime Minister, the move to reform and integrate childcare and education gathered pace. His personal commitment to bringing about the reforms was mentioned by several informants as being highly influential.

In March 1996, Persson announced that the whole system of early childhood and school-age childcare services – pre-schools, family daycare and free-time services – would be transferred to education: this was not to be a piecemeal reform, leaving the early years centres in social welfare while placing the pre-school class and school-age childcare within school. All were to come together under the auspices of education. The main planks supporting this decision were both economic and pedagogical. From the point of view of economics, he believed that to have provision for young children framed within education would promote a lifelong learning approach that was vital for Sweden's ability to compete as a 'knowledge society' in the world market. A recent report placed Sweden as 'the world's number one information economy', based on an index made up of telephone lines and mobile phones in use, computing and social infrastructure (Schofield, 2001, p 2). That this is a view shared at local level is evident from a quotation to be found in the education plan of one of the *communes* we studied:

> Today it is more important than ever to cultivate the human creative ability, because in the rapid changes we are experiencing it is only through creative imaginations and the power of initiative that individuals and society can adapt themselves to what is new and transform their reality.

At the same time, Persson valued the pedagogic developments that had taken place within the welfare system services. He believed that, within the education system, the influence of pre-schools and free-time services could spread to the school.

In 1996, the overall responsibility of the Ministry of Health and Welfare for pre-schools and free-time services was transferred to the Ministry of Education and Science. Administrative responsibilities passed, in 1998, from the National Board of Health and Social Welfare to the National Agency for Education, with responsibility for administration, monitoring standards, support and development across the system. This was not accomplished without some opposition from theoreticians, policy makers and practitioners, who were afraid that important pedagogical traditions would be lost or damaged and that a more instrumental approach to children and learning might be adopted within the formal education system. There was much discussion and publication as a result, including a document from the National Board of Health and Social Welfare celebrating the pedagogic approach that had been developed over many years in the pre-schools and free-time care services for which they had been responsible (Socialstyrelsen, 1997).

It should be emphasised that at this time of transfer certain important strategic goals for pre-schools and free-time services had largely been achieved, in particular an accessible service providing family support and promoting equal opportunities for men and women. This achievement was reflected in a 1995 law that entitled all working parents of children between one and 12 years of age, as well as parents of children with special needs, to a place in one of these services. Most *communes* were already able to meet this requirement.

In 1999, immediately after the transfer of government responsibility was completed, 75% of children aged from one to five years and 65% of children aged from six to nine years were in pre-schools or free-time services (Skolverket, 2000). Put another way, in the same year, 76% of one- to five-year-olds were in publicly funded services, mostly in pre-schools (65%), but some in family daycare (11%). Of the remaining children, half (11% of the total) were with parents taking parental leave (as were the great majority of children under one year of age), and 8% were cared for by employed (working shifts or at home) or unemployed parents, leaving just a handful (3%) with relatives or private family daycarers).

In short, the Swedish welfare system had succeeded in providing almost universal childcare for working parents. Now the focus could be on the child and on pedagogy. The Ministry of Education and Science was seen by many as the place to take forward this work, and as a fitting site for all services with a care and educational role.

More than one of our informants admired the stand the Prime Minister had taken and his vision for children and education. In many ways, he confronted the debate around the tensions between the traditions and values of the school and those of pre-school and free-time care services. More recently, with the reforms in place, he has spoken about the goals for the compulsory school being 'knowledge and love'. Informants commented on this choice of words with admiration. A senior civil servant commented that only he would have dared to use the word 'love' in this context and said that by 'love' he meant basic democratic values, safety, security and care – the basic human quality referred to by an informant quoted earlier.

But he was not alone in putting forward these views. A trades union official remarked that her union had published a paper with the same name and said that love was important because professionals should strive to connect with all children, who in turn should love to go to school. Other politicians had

Table 5.1: The number of children enrolled in care and education provision, 1996-2001

	Pre-school[a]	Pre-school class	Family daycare	Leisure-time centres	Total
1996	365,828	na	110,196	239,439	712,555
1999	318,660	112,251	69,300	332,168	832,379
2001	314,987	99,615	49,724	336,508	800,834
Net change in place 1996-2001	–50,841	na	–60,472	97,069	88,279
Percentage change in places 1996-2001	13.9	na	–54.9	40.5	12.4

Note:

[a] The introduction of the pre-school class in 1998 has entailed that the pre-school nowadays receives children aged between one and five, instead of one to six as before and that an increasing number of six-year-olds attend leisure-time centres. From 1998, the figures on the pre-school are not therefore directly comparable with figures from earlier years on daycare homes. Some caution should also be observed in making comparisons with previous years for leisure-time centres as well.

A further change is that from 1998 childcare statistics have been coordinated with school statistics with data presented from 15 October instead of 31 December as before.

Source: Skolverket

Table 5.2: Children enrolled in different types of childcare as a percentage of all children in the population in 1999 and 2001

		Proportion 1-5 years	Proportion 6-9 years	Proportion 10-12 years	Proportion 1-12 years
1999	Pre-school	63.8	0.9	na	21.6
	Leisure-time centres	0.3	62.2	6.6	2.3
	Family daycare	10.8	3.0	0.4	4.7
	Total	**74.9**	**66.1**	**7.0**	**49.3**
2001	Pre-school	67.8	0.6	na	22.8
	Leisure-time centres	0.2	66.1	8.3	24.9
	Family daycare	8.7	1.9	0.3	3.6
	Total	**76.7**	**68.6**	**8.6**	**51.3**
Percentage change 1999-2001		**1.8**	**2.5**	**1.6**	**2.0**

Source: Skolverket

shown commitment to change. Björn Flising notes that the Minister of Social Affairs, Ingela Thalén, had been instrumental in promoting children and child perspectives, as had the Minister of Schools, Ylva Johansson. Flising (2003) comments:

> She [Johansson] often started her speeches with the phrase 'for the children school shall be safe, joyful and promote learning – in this order'. In her work as minister she was a woman of fast actions and often quite outspoken. At a big conference in 1998, when the responsibility for pre-schools and school-age childcare was officially moved from the National Board of Health and Welfare to the National Agency for Education, Ylva Johansson said: 'Now it is very important that school does not seat its big ass down on pre-school and school-age childcare, but stands up in a meeting of mutual respect and joint responsibilities'.

So there was strong political support for the 'new' pedagogic approach and one that could put love, joy and safety alongside – and even ahead of – learning.

The incorporation of the pre-school class into the school

In 1998 it became mandatory for the *commune* to provide a pre-school class for six-year-olds, within the compulsory school. Compulsory school age remains seven years and, in theory, parents have the right to choose whether at age six children continue to attend a whole-day pre-school, separate from the compulsory school, or go to the pre-school class that is part of the school. In practice, however, the *commune* may not provide for six-year-olds in their pre-schools. So while it is not obligatory, almost all six-year-olds attend a pre-school class during school time *plus* school-based, school-age childcare services before and after school.

A more universal approach

The welfare services that now entered the educational domain had developed from what was largely targeted provision. It is true that the history of early years provision had also interwoven within it educational strands and emphases, with kindergarten experience long regarded as beneficial for children. But services had been provided at first for children seen as in need, and later for the children of working parents. Prior to the reforms discussed in this chapter, publicly provided and subsidised childcare was widespread, but it was not universally available as of right. However, since their move from welfare to education, Sweden has seen the development of childcare services into a genuinely universal service. In this they follow the pattern of the prime educational provision, state schooling, which had had a history of universal provision since the mid-19th century. It was, however, another 50 years before education was provided for all children. (We should point out that, while many welfare services had had quite elaborate educational content, schools had long sought to provide welfare measures as well as education. They had been a means of delivering a variety of resources for families, such as baths, free lunches and health services. They had been sites that could provide a means of influencing family behaviour: as one of our informants put it, a 'friendly control apparatus'.)

With education now taking responsibility for childcare, all children, irrespective of their parents' employment position, are entitled to attend a preschool for at least 15 hours a week from the age of 12 months. Before, a child could be denied a place, or lose an existing place, in a pre-school if his or her parents were not at work. Now provision has been extended, first to children of unemployed parents in 2001, then to children whose parents are on parental leave in 2002. Access to early childhood services has thus been disconnected from parents' labour market participation, with admission to provision becoming a child's right and pre-school attendance seen as of benefit to all.

This change in admission policy can be seen as substituting the principles of the education system for those of the welfare system. Further signs of this process can be seen with new legislation on parental fees (Regeringens proposition 1999/2000:129, Maxtaxa och allmän förskola m.m.). From 2003, all four- and five-year-olds are offered at least 525 hours per year of pre-school attendance free of charge. This is explicitly related to bringing pre-schools more into line with the principles of Swedish education: "[this change will] bring pre-school closer to the principle underlying all schools, that they should be free, available to all and provide equal services to all, a principle which, for schools at any rate, is now hardly questioned" (Regeringens proposition 1999/2000:129, Maxtaxa och allmän förskola m.m.).

Further, from 2002 *communes* have been recommended to set a ceiling on parental fees for services – both pre-schools and free-time services – that are not yet free. Fees for a first child in a pre-school should not be more than 3% of family income, with a maximum payment set at SEK1,140 (€123) per month; for free-time services, the recommended rates are 2% of income or SEK760 (€82) per month. Lower rates apply for subsequent children. *Communes* that adopt this recommendation will be compensated by central government for loss of revenue. By 2003 all *communes* had decided to take part in a system that had proved to be highly popular with the electorate.

These changes have been accompanied by further improvements in parental leave, which needs to be seen as closely coordinated with service provision: the right to a pre-school place starts from a child's first birthday, since it is assumed that parents will be taking paid leave before then. From 2002, the period of leave paid at 80% of earnings has been increased from 12 to 13 months, linked to extending that part of the leave that can be taken by either fathers or mothers (a policy intended to encourage take-up by men). Today, mothers and fathers each have a quota of two months' leave at high income-replacement rates, the remaining nine months to be divided between parents as they choose. At the same time as this change, an additional option for leave taking has been added, making it even more flexible: in addition to the existing options – to take leave on a full-time, half-time or quarter-time basis – it can now be taken one hour a day. Parents taking a part-time option can extend the period of leave accordingly.

The role of Skolverket

Since 1620, Sweden has separated central government from the civil service. This is reflected in the current structures of ministries and of national agencies. Today, the ministry responsible for all services is the Ministry of Education and Science, while *Skolverket* is the national agency that carries national policy forward, within a system that is, as we have seen, highly decentralised. The National Agency for Education has taken over the responsibilities for pre-schools and free-time services previously held by the National Agency for Health and Social Welfare. With the reforms, three members of staff transferred to *Skolverket*. It is a unitary service, not organised by type of service or by age group; there is, for example, no pre-school division.

Skolverket has an overview of how the system is working and the prevailing standards. *Communes* produce an annual review of their work for *Skolverket*, which so far does not include the work of pre-schools, although there is some discussion about whether this should be included.

A variety of methods has been used to monitor standards. For example, each year *Skolverket* has 'developmental dialogues' with some 20% of *communes* so that each *commune* is covered every five years. This project is intended to develop educational quality. The dialogue is based on the *commune's* review, any complaints received by *Skolverket* (for example, from parents), and *Skolverket's* analysis of statistics returned by the *communes*. During these dialogues, the team from *Skolverket* talks to various groups of professionals and members of the local community – but not very much with children.

In addition to looking at individual *communes*, *Skolverket* selects three topics of special relevance each year, such as local practice with slow learners, and visits some 20–25 *communes* to research these topics specifically. *Skolverket* is also about to start a project on first- and second-generation migrant children. The government may ask *Skolverket* to conduct specific studies; for example, the agency has produced work on a new type of school for six-year-olds. As well as this more consultative approach, *Skolverket* can investigate whether *communes* are complying with the law and regulations laid down at national level. Nevertheless, our informants told us that *Skolverket's* aim is to discuss with *communes* how they can improve on what they have achieved, and that the agency is much less interested in processes of inspection.

In 2003, *Skolverket* was reorganised and divided into two separate agencies: the National Agency for Education for more formal inspections, and the National Agency for School Improvement for school development.

Integration of services

We now turn to the ways in which bringing childcare and the pre-school class into the education system have been followed through, beyond administrative integration to the integration or coordination of many aspects of the various institutions involved, including most importantly the curriculum and staffing.

Integrated and coordinated curricula

In 1998, the curriculum for the compulsory school was amended to incorporate the pre-school class and the free-time service. The preamble to the curriculum also states that 'the pre-school class is the first step in implementing and fulfilling the goals of the curriculum. The leisure time centres [free-time services] should contribute to fulfilling these goals' (Swedish Ministry of Education and Science, 1998, p 1). The responsibility for the interpretation and realisation of the (very broad) curriculum goals was decentralised to the *communes* and thence to the schools. The new curriculum was much cited by those interviewed as influential and representing an integration beyond the merely administrative.

Also in 1998 came the publication of the first curriculum for the pre-school (Swedish Ministry of Education and Science, 1998). A senior civil servant and educationist told us that the pre-school curriculum had been very important for pre-school teachers and for parents. For both it had placed the pre-school firmly within the education system. Under the Ministry of Health and Welfare, there had been a curriculum – or at any rate an educational programme for pre-schools – but this had been guidance rather than a statutory instrument. Now the pre-school had its own curriculum, alongside curricula for the compulsory school and the non-compulsory upper secondary school. "The aim is that the three curricula should link into each other and take a common view of knowledge, development and learning".

The curriculum for the compulsory school system, the pre-school class and the leisure-time pedagogue sets two kinds of goals, goals to reach and goals to strive towards:

> Goals to strive towards indicate the direction of the work of the school.... Goals to reach express what the pupils at least shall have reached when they leave school. It is the responsibility of the school and the school head that the pupils are given the possibility to reach these goals. (Swedish Ministry of Education and Science, 1994, p 10)

The very nature of the curriculum allows for many decisions to be made by *communes* and by the school: a clear example of how power is decentralised to local level. The curricula are short, non-prescriptive documents of 22 pages in the case of the Curriculum for compulsory schools and of 16 pages for the Curriculum for the pre-school. The goals that are set are described in the broadest terms. There are also equally wide guidelines for staff as to how goals should be realised. The interpretation and realisation of the curricular goals are, in the first place, a matter for the *communes*, which formulate their own overall plans. Schools and pre-schools then work within the framework set by their own *commune*, formulating their own plans and goals.

Collaboration in practice

In practice, we found many signs of the cooperative approach that the integrated system sought to foster. In one *commune* we studied, we were told that the integration of pre-school, school, and free-time services allows the staff to talk of 'our children', with the teachers knowing the children in different settings and at different ages and stages of development, helping them to see the whole child. The official plan of a pre-school in another *commune* is shown in Box 5.4.

One dimension of service integration and continuity is often referred to by a commonplace Swedish metaphor: that of the 'red thread'. We were told that it comes from the practice of marking imported goods that had been cleared by customs with a red thread. The use of this expression implies activities that connect or continue over time. The expression has a positive connotation and is used with approval in order to describe the continuity of experience that the new system can produce for children.

For example, the expression was used in an all-age school for 900 pupils aged from six to 16 that we visited in central Sweden. The school's *rektor* was also responsible for two local pre-schools, so his position covered children and young people from one to 16 years of age. The school had two main sections within the same complex of buildings: the lower school for children aged from six to 12 years, which operated on the basis of four units, and a secondary school for 13- to 16-year-olds. There were four deputy heads. One of them, who worked across all the settings, had responsibility for the pre-schools, for the four school-age childcare *fritidshems* (one per unit), and for overseeing the

Box 5.3: Examples of curricular goals in the compulsory and pre-school curricula

Compulsory school goals:

History teaching should contribute to the pupils' assimilation of a cultural identity and provide a foundation for the pupils' desire to study, influence and develop society and its culture. The subject should also provide pupils with an instrument for developing an ability for critical thinking and an analytical approach.

In the subject areas of *sports and health* pupils have the opportunity to try and learn different games, dances, sports and to lead an active outdoor life. Games, dances and sports occur in similar forms all over the world and provide an important part of children's culture in all countries. Thus teaching the subject could contribute to strengthening the feeling of togetherness and develop understanding and respect for children with different backgrounds.

Social studies should contribute to obtaining pupils' knowledge about present conditions of society and social questions and their background and getting accustomed to searching for and assessing information. The task is also to give pictures of people in activities in different social contexts and in different parts of Sweden and other countries.

Teaching in *crafts* should give pupils knowledge of different methods within the area as well as materials, tools and machines and a feeling for aesthetic values. Craft studies should develop consciousness in the use of resources for consumption and production and make pupils aware of female and male traditions in crafts and also of the rich treasure of everyday life that is buried in these.

Pre-school curriculum goals:

The pre-school should try to ensure that children:
* feel a sense of participation in their own culture and develop a feeling and respect for other cultures;
* develop their motor skills, ability to coordinate, awareness of their own body, as well as an understanding of the importance of maintaining their own health and well-being;
* develop their ability to build, create and design using different materials and techniques.

educational ethos throughout the school. She had herself trained as a pre-school teacher. She said that she also saw herself as responsible for the 'red thread'. By this she meant that it was her responsibility to see that the different parts of the school – junior and secondary, the pre-school classes, school-age

Box 5.4: Collaboration with the school

We strive for a trusting collaboration with the school. We want to exchange information and experiences with the school's staff.

We want to find good routines to round off and finish the nursery school time. We have, after consultation with parents, 'handing over' talks with school staff before the start of school.

Children who require particular support should be noted and eventually a particular plan for the transition to school will be drawn up in collaboration with the school and parents.

We invite the school staff to the nursery, for example, for a drop-in, so that they get to know the children and parents.

We develop a sponsoring system ... so that the children get to know each other before starting school. We regularly visit the school.

The children go to school and have physical education classes during the spring term. They also eat in the school dining hall then and familiarise themselves with the outside environment of the school.

And a brochure produced by the *commune* where this pre-school was located says:

> In N [name of *commune*] we are proud of our schools – they have a fine reputation and their standards are a benchmark for other communities. This is partly due to the fact that N was the first Swedish municipality to introduce classes for six-year-olds.... We find solutions we believe in. Our pre-schools and primary schools are fully integrated. This holistic view means that our children enjoy an easier transition between the schools and classes. The many years of contact between staff and pupils make it possible to build rewarding and relaxed relationships between teachers, students and parents.

childcare, and the attached pre-schools – were coordinating their approaches to children so as to provide continuity for children from one year old up to 16 years old.

Staffing and teamwork

With the transfer of responsibility, the movement towards teamwork between teachers, pre-school teachers and free-time pedagogues continued to gather momentum. In many settings we saw staff teams, with members drawn from the different occupations, working together with groups of children – sometimes with the children organised on the basis of age, sometimes with children drawn from different age groups on the basis of ability. While overall responsibility for specific aspects of the work may lie with one team member, in practice team members plan and work together; for example, someone trained as a free-time pedagogue may work with children learning to read.

Cooperation is also valued for its own sake. A *commune* planning document stated:

> It is important that pupils have the opportunity to work in groups so that they can experience the knowledge and experience of their schoolmates. The adults must therefore, as role models, also carry out their tasks in varying types of teams. Group work for both adults and pupils, which means meeting both similarities and differences, is important for the development of learning.

A researcher told us that, where schools are working in a spirit of reform, they produce what looks like completely new practice. Different staff talk a lot together, discussing and planning work, valuing their own differing roles; children play, do a lot of experiments, sing and dance, work in different kinds of groups on themes that integrate different school subjects; and their use of time and space is more free-flowing than in traditional schools. (The same researcher had concerns that this was not always the case – as discussed later.)

Our local case studies also found regular meetings between teachers in different schools within the same *commune*, including both schools at primary and at secondary level.

The background and role of the rektor

Another feature of integration, and one that resonates with the recent Swedish reforms in teacher training (as discussed later), is that the school principal (*rektor*) may be drawn from any of the relevant professions – whether that of teacher in the compulsory school system, pre-school teacher or free-time pedagogue. Like the example above, in most *communes rektors* are responsible for clusters of schools, free-time services and pre-schools (as well as family daycarers). Again, this was seen as aiding integration, with one person responsible for the child's welfare and education from the age of one through to 16 years.

Rektors, whatever their professional backgrounds, have responsibility for teaching and the curriculum, as well as for what the curriculum calls 'pedagogic leadership', that is, having an overview of children's general welfare. Our informants told us that about half of all *rektors* had trained as pre-school teachers or free-time pedagogues. Broadening the background of *rektors* beyond school teaching was in itself seen as a means of bringing about greater integration between services. The professional backgrounds of *rektors* with pre-school or free-time training meant that they had been used to prioritising broad welfare issues in working with children and families. Especially important, they brought a more holistic pedagogy to their work – that is, they were used to considering the child as a whole person rather than focusing on their more cognitive attributes. Especially perhaps with the pre-school teachers, they came from a tradition that had developed its own understandings of 'learning' and of how and under what conditions children learn. This was wider than that of the more academic and formal understandings traditionally to be found in schools.

Both the reliance on teamwork, within schools and between services, and the appointment of non-teachers to the position of *rektor* indicate a reshaping of professional boundaries and identities, already in place at the time of national administrative integration.

However, teamwork, increased integration and professional cooperation can all highlight remaining differences between professions in terms of pay and conditions. There is some hierarchy in pay across occupations, from SEK15,500 (€1,674) a month for pre-school teachers and free-time pedagogues to SEK18,500 (€1,998) a month for a compulsory school teacher and SEK19,500 (€2,106) a month for a teacher in the upper secondary school – but these rates can vary. Pre-school teachers working in pre-schools have just two hours a week non-contact time; compulsory school teachers have about 10 hours a week. Differences remain, too, over annual leave. Schoolteachers have about 12 weeks' leave per year. Pre-school teachers and free-time pedagogues are entitled only to the same six weeks' annual leave as other working Swedes. They do not necessarily have time off during school holidays; on the contrary, they often have to work full-time providing childcare. Pre-school teachers in pre-school classes still may have 'employment with interruptions', meaning that, like schoolteachers, they leave their job when school is out for holidays, but, unlike schoolteachers, they also suffer an interruption or reduction in salary.

Staffing in the new system

A new and radical approach to professional education will, however, eventually blur existing divisions between staff still further or even do away with them entirely. A researcher, an expert in teacher education, told us that teacher education has been reformed every decade since 1954, and that this has always occurred a short time after school reforms. Teachers are educated, he said, with a particular model of the school in mind. The school that emerged in the late 1980s and throughout the 1990s was, as we have seen, a changing school and extended school, providing for children in new ways, taking the place of former services but beginning to draw on their traditions and pedagogies. What we have been describing so far is a new school. Some Swedish schools had in fact renamed themselves. As we wrote of earlier research:

> Elsewhere, we found institutions which were no longer called schools, but *houses*, incorporating as they did several functions and different professional groups working collaboratively. For example, there was *Emmahuset*, in

Gothenburg. The name was based on an acronym (MA) meaning the house of masses of activities. It served an area described as disadvantaged, where three quarters of the population were immigrants. Clusters of three classes, each for children of different ages, were grouped together and carried out many different activities with their teachers and their free-time pedagogues, who worked together as a team. The school's principal, whose background was as a free-time pedagogue, always referred to her institution as a House because its function was so much larger than that of a school, and the pedagogic approach to children's learning was different from that of the traditional school. (Moss and Petrie, 2002, p 158)

For some of our informants, as we shall see, the fear was always that the reforms might lead – or had led – to a diminution of pre-school and free-time traditions through the possibility of 'colonisation' by the school with its very different practices and discourses. However, one informant, while recognising that the school and pre-school operated with different discourses, had identified what the two traditions had in common: for example, a Swedish idea of democracy. She questioned the idea of proceeding by taking the best of the pre-school tradition and of the school and combining them, and moved instead to the idea of a new form of institution, a new meeting place, where both could bring their experience, deconstruct their old experience and build a new space for children and adults.

New spaces require new forms of professions. When they work together in teams, it is not always possible to distinguish the professional backgrounds of the different members of staff – in some ways a new profession of children's worker was emerging. The discussion that accompanied the reforms had often been concerned with the nature of this profession and how it might best be constructed, supported and named. We were told that there was strong support in some quarters for teachers, pre-school teachers and free-time pedagogues all to be known as 'pedagogues', so that the breadth of their work would be encompassed and the traditions of the pre-school and the free-time care service would not be lost but would further influence the more formal proceedings of the compulsory school.

These arguments did not hold sway, however. The teachers' union (*Lärarförbundet*) believed that the term 'teacher' denoted a higher status than 'pedagogue'. More recent events have led to all these professions being conceptualised as teachers and with joint training and education (as discussed later). The discussion continues, however, in other forms. These are teachers who are not conceived of in narrowly educational terms. In Sweden, education is itself seen as one aspect of public welfare. For example, an expert commission on welfare set up by the Swedish government after the 1998 election adopted a wide perspective covering health, schools, childcare and eldercare. A government committee is now looking at the vocabulary in use in different parts of the educational system, which indicates different emphases and contrasting interests emanating from different professional groups. For example, the use of words such as 'pupils', 'teachers' and 'education' may be seen as belonging more to the school than 'children', 'pedagogues' and 'pedagogy', terms that are commonly used in pre-school and free-time services. Some informants reported that '*utbildning*' (broadly, education that considers the child holistically) is more capable of encapsulating the field than '*Schoolform*', which relates more to schooling. Also, while all staff are to be known as teachers, there remains the question of how children should be constructed within the new schools: should they be referred to as pupils or children or by some other name? An informant from one of the trades unions said that, while the commission was prepared for all staff to be seen as teachers, it is not comfortable with seeing the youngest children (from one year old) as 'pupils'.

Integrated teacher training

One informant told us that teacher education is the engine by which politicians can drive school reform and reorganisation. The reform of qualification and education for the professionals involved is as far-reaching as the reforms outlined above. A new integrated system of teacher training was introduced in 2001, replacing eight of the 11 degrees that provided university-level qualifications for staff in pre-schools, schools and free-time services. In this new system, there will be one profession – a new form of teacher – rather than three separate professions of pre-school teacher, free-time pedagogues and compulsory schoolteacher.

Some staff have lower levels of qualification, including assistants working in pre-schools with a qualification obtained in the upper secondary school. But, in 1999, 53% of pre-school staff and 63% of free-time service workers had

Table 5.3: The number of employees in pre-school and free-time centres, by qualification in 2001 (expressed as proportion of staff in brackets)

Qualification	Pre-school	Free-time centre
Pre-school teacher	29,855 (50.9)	4,859 (25.1)
Free-time pedagogue	337 (0.6)	5,845 (30.2)
Teacher training	299 (0.5)	357 (1.8)
Childminder/childcare worker[a]	25,191 (42.9)	na
Youth recreation leader	79 (0.1)	669 (3.5)
Other training for work with children[a]	804 (1.4)	na
No childcare training	2,138 (3.6)	na
No information		7,649 (39.5)
Total	**58,689**	**19,379**

Note: [a]Due to new collection procedures for employees in leisure-time centres, information on qualification is collected almost solely from the higher education register. Childminder and childcare courses are largely taken by 16- to 19-year-olds in the upper secondary school and are not included in this register, which means that information about qualification is lacking for these persons.

Source: Skolverket (2001b)

professional qualifications. With the introduction of the pre-school curriculum and its emphasis on pedagogy, most municipalities have decided to decrease the number of assistants in favour of more qualified teachers or pedagogues, while training for assistants no longer exists.

To qualify as a teacher in the new training system, whether for a professional post in a pre-school, a pre-school class, a free-time service or the first years of compulsory school, 140 credits are required. One credit is obtained through one week of study, so that one academic year provides 40 credits. In order to work in the higher levels of compulsory school or in the upper secondary school (for 16- to 19-year-olds), 180 credits are required, although for some specialisms up to 220 credits are necessary.

A central feature of the new system is that all teachers will be required to obtain 60 credits, involving a year-and-a-half's study, in the general area of teaching. This provides a common core for all school staff, whether they intend to teach in pre-school or in the upper secondary school. Not only are all students studying the same central courses over the first years of their training, they are also studying together, in whatever field they eventually work.

In addition, students must obtain credits that relate to particular professional orientations, for example, to the age group or setting (including free-time services) that best fits their professional aspirations. This is in order to develop professional competency. They are also required to deepen one specific educational area, which might be science, social studies or a practical or aesthetic subject. The combination of specialisms gives each student, on graduation, a distinctive profile or professional orientation.

We interviewed staff at two institutions where teachers were trained, and the following main themes emerged from the interviews:

- The integration of training and education would provide a common status, a common knowledge base and a common professional identity for staff across the education system. The common core of subjects, which are to be studied by all students whether their interests lie in teaching physics to 16- to 19-year-olds in teaching music in the first years of compulsory school, or in school-age childcare especially, is intended to unite the profession.
- Under the new system, former professional labels will be less applicable or, in the view of some interviewees, inapplicable. Even though some teachers might choose to work in, say, a pre-school rather than elsewhere in the system, they would be first and foremost teachers, not teachers of a certain age group or of a certain subject, but with a professional orientation (*inrikting*) towards different ages or subjects.
- Because the professional divides are confronted, teachers know where children are going to in the school system and where they have come from. It will make for a more open-minded profession.
- While training within subject areas, especially for teachers in secondary and upper secondary schools, had always been strongly specialist, now all teachers would have a specialist knowledge base. Educating children for today's

Box 5.5: An excerpt from the University of Gothenburg's teacher education curriculum for 2002 (translated by the research team)

The general area of teaching (GAT) is compulsory for all prospective teachers and encompasses 60 credits, 16 of which are activity-based training (practice placements). It deals with areas of knowledge that are important for all teachers regardless of which activity the pedagogical competency will be used for. GAT is made up of two main types of course, equal in scope:

• Courses that deal with issues of learning, instruction and remedial teaching, socialisation, culture and society as well as the school's social task, democracy and value basis.

• Multidisciplinary subject courses whose content is made up of several different subject areas. Their purpose is to provide perspective in those areas of knowledge that teachers work with and provide a basis for choosing and organising the content of the pedagogical activity.

GAT offers the students the chance to develop a knowledge basis for pedagogical work and acquire different perspectives on teaching and teaching conditions. It also gives them the chance to develop various competencies in advance of becoming teachers, such as creating encounters that are pedagogical, learning to be inspiring teachers, learning how knowledge and learning vary in time and space and achieving learning environments for all children and young adults. The students also have the chance to develop, over time, the ability to create professional, social and cultural interactions in pedagogical work.

world requires this. Children ask demanding questions about the world around them and they should have access to informed adults.

• If teachers are educated together, they can teach together, in teams, bringing different subject specialisms to the team; they are better prepared to work collaboratively. Teamwork will become especially important. Because Swedish teachers would be expert in specific areas of knowledge they would have to learn to collaborate. A student's choice of courses and of practice placements would produce a specific profile. In recruiting staff, school principals would need to choose according to their requirements and think in terms of building a team of teachers with a range of profiles that met the school's needs.

To return to the point made earlier, although the term 'teacher' was chosen to describe the work of these variously specialist professionals, their role as pedagogues was explicitly acknowledged by some of the informants. As we were told by one informant who had been deeply involved in designing the new Swedish system, students start with a 10-week course on learning in which they look not only at learning as a subject and their own learning strategies, but also at themselves as learning persons and about their own values. He said that the most important thing is to understand how children learn about democracy, about their own behaviour and about values. 'We're pedagogues, all of us', he said. But with most new students seeing themselves as, for example, high-school mathematics teachers at the end of course, it would take a while to bring them round to being pedagogues. These tensions were reported as being mirrored in teacher training institutions, between academics in specialist subjects – for example, in the mathematics faculty of a university, who were said to see teachers as carrying knowledge from the university into the school system – and staff in teacher education who were more interested in the pedagogical processes involved.

We carried out our research in the first year of these reforms, which had been introduced with great speed and, some said, with little time for preparation. It was too early to expect a realistic, critical appraisal of them. The first graduates from the new system will enter work in 2004.

The extent of integration

In summary, it may be seen that in Sweden the integration of early childhood services, school-age childcare services and schooling has been thorough, extending well beyond the administrative, with the intention of:

- integrating the curricula of the compulsory school, the pre-school class and the free-time care service;
- coordinating the curricula of the pre-school and the upper secondary school with the curriculum of the compulsory school, the pre-school class and the free-time care service;
- integrating the child and young person's experience across time, between – for example, pre-school, pre-school class and school, and lower secondary and upper secondary school – by means of:
  ‣ coordinated or integrated curricula;
  ‣ the one and a half years of teacher training in core educational subjects, required in common for all practitioners;
  ‣ constructing the professionals across all these settings as teachers;
- integrating the child's day, physically, with care and schooling/pre-schooling taking place in the same setting and staff working in teams (for children aged from six to 10 years and older in some schools); and
- integrating the child's day, at the level of pedagogy, by means of the common curriculum and because they meet the same staff within the same setting.

Relations with other services

With the reforms must come some readjustment in the relationships of the ministries, agencies and services concerned. We provide a short account of these because they are of relevance to the somewhat critical evaluation of the reforms that some of our interviewees produced.

Social welfare

With pre-school and free-time services now placed in the Ministry of Education and Science, the Ministry of Health and Social Affairs is no longer responsible for universal welfare services for children and families. Our interview with officials at the ministry seemed to suggest that history had moved on very quickly from the days when they had responsibility for these early childhood and school-age childcare services and that these services were no longer of particular interest to them. In part this may have been due to the transfer of staff with relevant expertise to the Ministry of Education and Science.

The Ministry of Health and Social Affairs retains responsibility for targeted services, such as adoption, looked-after children and supportive case work. It is also responsible for parental leave policy as well as for overseeing all policy proposals that concern children. These are sent to the Children's Policies Coordination Unit of the Ministry of Health and Social Affairs, which has to look at whether proposals accommodate the child's perspective and conform to the UN Convention on the Rights of the Child. The ministry is responsible for the implementation and coordination of the Convention at national level by all ministries, national boards and agencies. On these matters it also collaborates with the Children's Ombudsman.

At local level, certain social welfare services may be incorporated within the school. For example, all schools should have a school nurse who visits, for example, two or three days a week. The remit of the nurse goes beyond developmental checks and help with minor illnesses to include being available for children to discuss any worries and to offer support. This latter role may also be taken by a social worker or counsellor (*kurator*). There is no national requirement that schools have such a post but many do, if only on the basis of two or three days a week. *Kurators* usually work only in secondary and upper secondary schools. Nurses and *kurators* may be managed by the *commune* centrally, but they also form part of a school's welfare system and are a resource for school staff as well as for children. In one *commune* we visited, they were also coordinated with the *commune's* psychology and special needs services, within the education department. In contrast, in another *commune* we visited *kurators* and field social workers in contact with children and families who all came under one unified welfare and education department. Different *communes* organise their departments in different combinations.

There was some evidence of problems about the boundaries between school welfare staff and *commune* social worker staff: who was responsible for what?

The cultures of the two sorts of services were also said to differ, with educational welfare staff being perceived as more 'child-centred' and social services more 'family-centred'.

More adults in school

Our informants provided evidence that the school was developing its welfare base through a new policy towards getting more adults, apart from the professional teachers, into the schools. One interviewee told us that in the 1960s and 1970s many new professionals had come into the schools, supplementing or complementing the role of teachers. These had included psychologists and counsellors. There had also been a place for 'student assistants', often people waiting to undertake qualification who could, for example, help supervise children during the lunch break. However, the recession of the 1990s with its resultant economic pressures led to less essential staff (in school education terms) being cut back.

At the time of our interviews, with an improved economy Sweden was looking to put more adults back into the schools: SEK17 billion (€1.8 billion) was available for the *communes* for additional adults to be employed in schools and *communes* had to show that the number of adults in schools had increased. We were told that schools and *communes* would be looking at alternative resources to implement this policy. For example, they might recruit people from minority ethnic groups who, although not professionally qualified, might be more capable of communicating with members of the local community and perhaps with children. They could be seen as cultural assistants who bridged Swedish and other cultures. Such people might have a different relationship with children from that of teachers and, without formal teaching responsibilities, could have more time than the teacher as an additional person for the children to relate to.

The school is obliged to provide Swedish language lessons for those children who do not speak Swedish, as well as mother-tongue lessons. It is not obligatory for the children to take part in these lessons. Somewhat more than half of those entitled to this language support use it. Pre-schools are supposed to support the child's development of her or his mother tongue, but there are no regulations concerning this matter. Some 50 *communes* offer mother-tongue training in their pre-schools but at the national level only 13% of children at pre-schools with a mother tongue other than Swedish take part (Skolverket, 2003).

The Family Resource Centre

A somewhat new organisational model for the youngest children (babies and toddlers) is the neighbourhood-based Family Resource Centre, which has been introduced in an increasing number of municipalities, especially in culturally mixed areas with large numbers of minority ethnic families. This more targeted provision represents a slight shift in policy. As one informant (the head of a local joint social services and education agency) told us, while services were good at the universal level – for example, school nurses, child and maternal health services – Sweden could be seen as less good with 'at risk' groups. In part this was because, with the low level of child poverty and good universal services, fewer children were 'at risk'. In addition, this informant said that Sweden did not wish to label children in terms of risk factors – but these sometimes needed to be addressed.

At the heart of the Family Resource Centre is the *öppen förskola* (open pre-school), where parents can drop in with their children but have to remain with them, and cannot leave them in the care of the pre-school teacher. The open pre-school, which can exist independently, is in this case the hub for other child health and care services. Here, the pre-school teacher and other professional staff are available for casual contact and advice. We were told that evaluations conducted at the University of Gothenburg show they are valuable services. However, it is possible that the universalisation of pre-school services (as discussed earlier) that has arisen in the wake of their coming under the Ministry of Education and Science might result in more parents preferring to use the public pre-schools rather than these specially targeted centres. Also, with fees set at no more than 1-3% of family income, and with unemployed parents and those on parental leave now entitled to a place, there is some financial pressure on the *communes* to maximise the use of mainstream services. This may mean that the *communes* can no longer afford open pre-schools, and may see less need for them – and the same may hold for the special pre-schools for children for whom Swedish is not their first language. Just as with special education, in which supported provision within mainstream services is a goal that is by and large achieved, the foothold of separate provision is not very secure where universal services are the norm.

Leisure services

The pedagogical responsibilities of the *commune* are not confined to its provision of schools and welfare measures, but can be exercised through a rich programme of classes, clubs and events, coordinated to greater and lesser extents with the school and education.

For example, in a *commune* that was one of our case studies, with a population of around 50,000 people, leisure – or free-time – activities for children and young people outside of school-age childcare included:

- outreach to newborn children and their parents, from the library service;
- 400 sports clubs;
- a dance pedagogue and an arts pedagogue, based in the *commune* arts centre, who worked full-time with children both through the schools and outside school;
- youth clubs;
- youth cafes (for disadvantaged young people);

- youth events such as a pop concert and the annual youth festival for school leavers; and
- various music and dance classes and schools.

Concerns about the reforms

In this section, we consider some of the concerns expressed by those we interviewed about the reforms and how they were progressing. Most, perhaps all, of our informants seemed pleased with the spirit of the reforms and enthusiastic about their potential. Nevertheless this approval was sometimes expressed alongside some qualifications as to how things were working out, or concerns about future developments. The new central position of the school, given its traditional ways of working and of conceptualising children, was challenging for some informants, alongside anxieties about the way in which school-age childcare and the pre-school class were developing and about continuing inequalities between staff.

'Schoolification'

A term that was used quite frequently by our informants was that of the 'schoolification' of the services that had come into the education system. When interviewees used the term they were suggesting a demotion of the culture of pre-school classes and free-time services and of their staff. Yet the intention of the reforms had been to reform the school. Introducing the ethos and traditions of the other services, with the coming together of the three different professions, had been seen as having great potential to create new approaches. A researcher told us that, instead, there was evidence in the pre-school class of a move to more subject-oriented approaches, and the introduction of temporal and spatial divisions (such as fixed timetable periods and designated spaces for work), although there were considerable variations between schools. A director of education of one of our case study *communes* believed that the pre-school had become more like the traditional school, with staff concentrating more on teaching children rather than employing the pedagogies developed in the pre-school and free-time care services.

Someone who trained free-time pedagogues was "not convinced about 'learning' being the be all and end all" of provision, because children do not construct their experience in terms of learning. Nevertheless, she reported that free-time pedagogues had been heard to ask children what they had learned in an activity. This informant feared that the stress on learning meant that the traditional way of working was threatened, adding: "Sitting round an open fire together is important, friends are important and, for everyone, existing is important, and being. Learning is just *one* theoretical way of constructing life. The hands, the heart and the head (*must all be addressed*) – but the heart can be forgotten".

Also, while many respondents referred to an increase in team working since the reforms were implemented, the teacher was often seen as the leader of the team, while the other staff were there to assist. One free-time pedagogue referred to her role in the classroom as working with the class teacher and helping with more practical tasks such as baking and drawing but definitely not teaching. In similar vein, some fear was expressed that the new system of teacher education would mean fewer students training for the pre-school and free-time care services because of ongoing pay and status differentials within the system: given the opportunity to choose where to specialise after starting a course, too many students might opt for schoolteaching.

A researcher who was well placed to comment on the process of the reforms believed that they had a strong developmental potential but that this could be realised only if certain prerequisites were met. These included sufficient time and resources to implement the reform throughout the whole of the local *commune* organisation, including politicians, managers and practitioners. Currently, there was insufficient support for planning or reflection, for opportunities to internalise the new ideas in the curriculum, or for the development of an adequate theoretical framework to give them tools (Skolverket, 2001a).

A three-year project conducted by *Skolverket* studied different aspects of integration between pre-school classes (six-year-olds), compulsory school for younger children (seven- to nine-year-olds) and free-time services. They found risks of, and strong tendencies for, the dominance of school culture and school codes, rather than the three parts developing new perspectives and working methods. This 'schoolification' also held for the work in mixed team groups, in which the schoolteacher often took a leading role and pre-school teachers and free-time pedagogues often took the role of assistant to the schoolteacher. It was also not unusual for them to adopt the perspectives and aims of the schoolteacher and to develop their own work in this way.

Other reasons for lack of progress that other informants cited included: teaching staff who were resistant or opposed to change and who wished to continue with more formal and autonomous methods of working with children; pre-school teachers and free-time pedagogues who were over-impressed by the role of the teacher, whose practice they might try to emulate; the influence of national goals and grades; and the increasingly important subject base of schooling with a gradual introduction of school subjects from the pre-school (where there has been little subject-based learning) to the secondary school (where pupils have a curriculum of 16 or 17 subjects).

Yet one informant, a researcher working on different aspects of the reform of teacher training, told us that some emerging research painted a more optimistic picture. He said that, while the traditional school culture recognises the professional competencies of others and proclaims that all professionals working with children are equal, nevertheless, just as in Orwell's *Animal farm*, "all animals are equal but the pigs are a little more equal", so teachers are a little 'more equal' than others. However, over the course of three years he had seen teachers slowly moving away from a mechanistic model of teaching and learning, and claimed that teachers working within compulsory schools had learned to talk *with* children, not *to* children, which is the norm in the school tradition. The pedagogues have brought with them a different conception of the child and the teachers have learned from this.

Two other points were made as to how the reforms have affected children. First, according to an informant who is responsible for the training of free-time pedagogues, an unintended result of bringing six-year-olds into school was an adverse effect on the development of school-age childcare. Staff are very aware of the needs of the youngest children, who are now aged six years rather than seven years. This has had a great impact on the activities undertaken in free-time care services, making them much less attractive for children aged nine to 12 years, who are entitled to attend but now are less likely to do so. Second, from their fourth year in school, when children are aged 10 or 11 years, groups of children are reorganised into new classes. These classes (grades four to six) are usually staffed only by those whose training has been as schoolteachers: there are no pre-school teachers, and free-time pedagogues are rarely found in the teams of staff. Therefore, the pedagogy with which the children have engaged in their earlier school careers is disrupted. An administrator, working in a *commune*, told us that there needs to be a professional team that shares understandings of knowledge and learning throughout education. At present, teachers in grades four to six may feel that teachers working with lower grades have prepared children too little for subject- and goal-focused work. This is still more apparent when the children reach grades seven to nine, in which teachers are often much more subject-oriented than are their colleagues who work with younger children. These problems of professional and pedagogic discontinuity are among those that the reformed system of teacher education seeks to address, with its common core education for all professionals.

The place of the upper secondary school

A few informants drew our attention to the somewhat anomalous position of the upper secondary school for 16- to 19-year-olds. They believed that the integration that has so far been achieved between the compulsory school and other services needed to extend to these schools, which were operating separately from the rest of the system, in terms of both management and pedagogy, and had been little influenced by the reforms. In one of the *commune*s studied, a local politician said that it would be good to have the schools organised for people aged one to 20 without any gaps between the different parts of the system.

Observations

This chapter has described how, over the course of a little more than a decade, from the late 1980s to the early years of the 21st century, Sweden reformed its education system, enlarging its remit so as to cover services previously regarded as within the province of welfare. Today, the Swedish childcare and education system is governed by a single government department, and a single agency is responsible for its administration, its monitoring, support and development. Integration first started in the *communes*, to which decision-making powers had been devolved in the early 1990s. Services are funded and, for the most part, provided by *communes* on the basis of central government grants and, in the case of pre-schools and free-time services, a low-level parental contribution. So, while there is some (state-funded) independent provision, most provision across early childhood and school-age childcare services, as well as schools, has one local provider and one local administrative system. There are also various parents' and students' boards that, potentially, have an input into the school's organisation and into matters concerning standards. Importantly, a government agency, *Skolverket*, monitors the standards achieved in the *communes* and engages in developmental dialogues with them in order to bring about improvements and to maintain equal standards across the national system.

As a result of the reforms, children can now experience an integrated school day, with education and care in one setting and an integrated educational career from age one to age 16 – although it seems that there is still work to be done to integrate schooling for older children and young people fully into the system. Teamwork between the various professionals (teachers, free-time pedagogues and pre-school teachers) is used as the basis for a more integrated experience for children, both over the years and in the course of the hours they spend in school premises each day. The curricula of the various services that form the education system have either been integrated or (for both the pre-school and the upper secondary school) coordinated with each other.

The newly integrated teacher education for all teachers in the compulsory school and the upper secondary school and all (in current terms) pre-school teachers and free-time pedagogues is a far-reaching step. It is seen by some as the means to achieve, eventually, a desired model of school, a new form of school, that serves many functions, with teams of staff who, while capable of carrying out different functions and expert in different areas, share a common core of pedagogic knowledge and values.

In part, these measures have been informed by a pragmatic approach to financial constraints. But we were also impressed by how the history of integration reveals an ongoing debate about the place of the child in society, and the sort of learning and knowledge that is needed in today's world. If it is the case that "public provisions for children are inextricably linked with how we understand childhood and our image of the child" (Moss and Petrie, 2002, p 2), then the Swedish child that emerges from interviews, case studies and the perusal of documents was a strong child, responsible and independent, a co-constructor of knowledge alongside adults.

The universal orientation of the Swedish welfare system and the broad concept of pedagogy has facilitated extensive integration of former welfare services into the education system. This has been further facilitated by an awareness of the need for change in schools and schoolteaching. The idea of finding a 'new meeting place' where these different services can forge new relationships and practices provides a strong metaphor for the changes that many seek, although colonisation or 'schoolification' remains a widespread concern. Taking early childhood and school-age childcare services into education has been accompanied by a policy to cut the link between access to certain services and parental employment: services are available as of right to all children and the focus is now on children and their appropriate pedagogies rather than on working parents – whose needs are seen, largely, as already met. In the Swedish context, universal educational services are seen broadly as having a welfare function, which raises questions about the role and viability of more targeted services.

Part Three:
A comparative overview and future directions

SIX

Cross-national comparisons

Having looked at each of our three countries individually, we turn now to comparing the different national experiences. What has merging departmental responsibility for childcare and education, pre-school and school actually meant in terms of policy, provision and practice? How can we characterise the 'integration' process in each case? How far has integration gone and what dimensions are involved? How can we make sense of the different experiences? How do they relate, for example, to the contextual issues we outlined in Chapter Two? We hope that this comparative process will enable us not only to conclude that there are differences between the three countries, but also to prepare the ground for defining some critical questions for the future direction of children's services, the subject of our final chapter.

In this chapter, we begin by comparing the extent and nature of integration across the three countries, both structurally and conceptually. We then consider the relationships both between the three services on which we have focused – early childhood education and care, compulsory schooling and school-age childcare – and between them and other services for children and families. We conclude that the integration process was fundamentally different in Sweden from that in England and Scotland, and end the chapter by considering the difference and the reasons for it.

The nature and extent of integration: structures

Our starting point was a similar reform in England, Scotland and Sweden: departmental reorganisation at national level that brought together responsibility for early childhood education and care, compulsory schooling and school-age childcare. In all three countries, this involved a transfer of responsibility for some services from welfare to education departments. But, behind this superficial similarity, important national differences are apparent.

In Sweden, the transfer involved the whole system of early childhood education and care ('pre-schools' and family daycare for children up to school age) together with school-age childcare. In England and Scotland, where responsibility for early childhood education and care had always been split, the transfer involved moving that part ('daycare') that was located in welfare. In Scotland, the process of departmental reform also included bringing child welfare and family support services into the Scottish Executive Education Department, to create a broader remit for children and families than in either England or Sweden (although England has very recently followed suit with the establishment of a Minister for Children, Young People and Families in the DfES whose remit includes child welfare and family support).

In England, departmental integration did not immediately mean organisational integration of early education and childcare: although within one department, initially they remained divided between different departmental sections. But, at the time that full organisational integration did finally occur, with childcare and education coming together within one unit, departmental responsibility for that unit was once again split. In five years, therefore, England had moved from welfare and education dividing responsibility for early education and childcare, to education having sole responsibility, to employment and education sharing responsibility through a single administrative unit.

In all three countries, local authorities led the way on departmental integration of childcare and early years education with compulsory education, although local integration of responsibility was more widespread in Sweden and in Scotland than in England prior to national-level change. Some local authorities in all three countries had gone further, bringing child welfare and, in some cases, other services (for children but also on occasion for adults too) within the same department as early childhood services, schools and school-age childcare.

Despite this 'vanguard' role of local authorities in all three countries, the relationship between national and local government is very different in Sweden from that in Scotland and, particularly, England. Over the past 20 years, Swedish local authorities (*communes*) have become more powerful as responsibilities, including schools, have been decentralised by national government. *Communes* remain the main providers of services. The national regulatory system – in which we include curricula, standards, inspection and child assessment – is light, leaving much to local interpretation and decision. All this is in marked contrast to England, where local authorities themselves now provide few services and national government has a direct relationship with individual childcare services and schools, and operates a centralised and prescriptive system of policy direction, service regulation and evaluation. In Scotland, government is a good deal more directive than in Sweden, though less so than in England; local authorities have somewhat greater control over funding than is evident in England and are somewhat more visible in the provision of services.

The structure of services is also very different between Sweden on the one hand and England and Scotland on the other. Prior to departmental integration, Sweden had a rather uniform and integrated system of services, in terms not only of providers (mostly *communes*) but also types of provision. Most children below six years of age who were not cared for at home by parents attended 'age-integrated' centres – pre-schools – open all day and all year and combining, in UK terms, 'care' and 'education'; nearly all of the remainder were at family daycarers, employed by *communes*. Pre-schools were the product of the full integration, in the 1960s and 1970s, of two different services: part-time kindergartens and full-time daycare (Lenz Taguchi and Munkammer, 2003). So, for many years before the transfer of responsibility to education, pre-schools had been the backbone of Swedish early childhood services, the basis on which provision was expanded from the late 1960s.

In the 1990s, a new type of integrated provision began to emerge. The 'whole-day school' combined a new form of provision, the pre-school class for six-year-olds, with compulsory schooling and school-age childcare services – although the extent of integration between the services and their workers varied from school to school. Departmental integration in Sweden, therefore, has led to few changes in the structure of services, which were already integrated or integrating around two institutions: the pre-school and the school.

Without a strong public policy interest, as in Sweden, the period from the 1960s in England and Scotland saw increasingly fragmented early childhood services. School-based nursery classes grew, but insufficiently to meet demand and with much variation in levels of provision between local authorities; playgroups and (in England) reception classes expanded to fill the gap. Family centres emerged in the 1980s to provide family support and community development. From the late 1980s (in England) and through the 1990s, there was a dramatic growth in private nurseries, catering for working parents and surpassing in the number of places the previous mainstay of formal 'childcare', childminders. During the 1990s, school-age childcare services began to expand, from a low base, located sometimes in schools, sometimes elsewhere.

Unlike Sweden, therefore, the legacy inherited by the reform process in England and Scotland was a diversity of services and providers: what some might term a mixed economy, others might call a fragmented muddle in which different providers and services targeted different children and pursued different purposes. Some initiatives have been taken post-1997 to create more integrated services. In the early childhood field this has mainly been in England and involves Early Excellence Centres and the recently proposed Children's Centres. However, these are not widespread: the former consisted essentially of a handful of demonstration projects while the latter, when open, will be confined to 'disadvantaged areas'. Most provision will continue, as before, to be fragmented, different types offering different services on different conditions to different children and families, each type dominated by a different type of provider.

For older children post-1997, school-age childcare services have increased rapidly, many funded initially (but not in the long term) by lottery money. While much of this provision has been in schools, it has not been part of schools. More innovatively, there has been some rethinking of the school and its role. Scotland has led the way here, with New Community Schools and a National Debate on Education. England in 2003, with its extended schools initiative just beginning in selected areas, was where Scotland was in 1997 with its pilot New (now Integrated) Community Schools.

We can see here examples of a major difference between Sweden, England and Scotland, a difference we shall explore and illustrate further as we proceed. Early childhood education and care services in Sweden have long been fully integrated; the move to the whole-day school points towards a further merging of previously separate services. The move to new community or extended schools in Scotland and England represents an attempt to better link – 'join up' – a range of distinct services so they can more effectively tackle a range of social problems. But neither here nor in early childhood services is there evidence of widespread integration of previously separate services where integration is understood as merging or fusion.

In Sweden, the same process of structural integration is apparent in the workforce, but in this case following, not preceding, the transfer of departmental responsibilities. Prior to departmental integration, the Swedish workforce in early childhood services, schools and school-age childcare was divided between three main occupations. However, the divisions were already bridged to a certain extent, unlike in England and Scotland. All three occupations were trained at a higher education level, even if on separate courses of somewhat different lengths. In schools, teamworking involving all three occupations had been developing alongside the emergence of the whole-day school. *Rektors*, who could come from any of the three occupations, were managing clusters of services. Workers from the three occupations were members of the same trade union, following a merger of unions in 1991 – with union membership overall very high. Teachers enjoyed better pay and other employment conditions, but the differential was not that large – and the great majority of workers in all three occupations were employed by *communes* after the delegation of responsibility for employing teachers from central government to *communes*. These conditions were all favourable to the most momentous move in the Swedish reform process since departmental integration: the introduction of an integrated training system leading to a new teaching qualification, encompassing the former three separate occupations.

By contrast, in England and Scotland the division between childcare workers and teachers before departmental integration was wide and unbridged. It included large differences in training, pay, type of employer and union membership. Since departmental integration, there has been no question of merging these two workforces: it has never appeared on the policy agenda. It is inconceivable in England and Scotland for a nursery or school-age childcare worker to be appointed to manage a school, as happens in Sweden. Not least of the problems of attempting to integrate occupations would be the large gap in training and pay, with private childcare providers unable to improve workforce conditions significantly without charging parents substantially more: most, if not all, providers simply see higher fees as a non-starter. Instead, measures since departmental integration have focused on improving training opportunities for childcare workers, on making it easier to move either within childcare work or from being a childcare worker to being a teacher: they have been essentially incremental rather than restructuring.

At the same time, a further division in the workforce has become increasingly apparent. Within English and Scottish schools post-1997, there has been a large increase in assistants, who can be seen as forming a third distinct group in the workforce, closer to childcare workers than to teachers in terms of pay and training. Staffing in English and Scottish schools is increasingly differentiated and hierarchical, with teachers supported by swelling numbers of assistants (with a 'higher-level' assistant proposed for England), while in many schools a separate group of childcare workers staff on-site school-age childcare services.

Swedish schools, by contrast, incorporate school-age childcare services. These 'whole-day schools' are staffed by teams of professional workers, whose members are now beginning to receive a common training leading to a common qualification, although with the potential for a wide range of more specialised interests and expertise among team members. Assistants in schools are uncommon, and are dwindling in pre-schools. While there has been a move to increase the number of adults in school, these are seen as bringing in a range of community resources rather than as quasi-professionals or assistants to professionals.

There are, however, some interesting similarities in workforce development. In both Scotland and Sweden, new types of cross-service manager are emerging to support closer relationships between services. The Scottish New Community Schools initiative, intended to offer a more integrated approach to education, health and family support, has introduced new posts to support connections between services: 'integration manager' (or equivalent) posts have been established in many areas, while Glasgow has clustered nursery, primary and secondary schools into 'learning communities', each with a lead principal who can come from any level of school. In Sweden, the *rektor* has responsibility for a cluster of different services, from family daycare through to schools and from pre-schools to clubs for teenagers.

Two other features are important in assessing the extent and nature of structural reform. First, funding. Before departmental integration in 1996, all Swedish services were mainly or wholly publicly funded on the basis of supply subsidy, that is, direct funding of services. The main difference was that services then in the education system – schools – were completely free to parents at the time of use; while parents were expected to pay fees for all services in the welfare system – pre-schools and free-time care services – although the fees accounted for less than a fifth of total costs. The funding difference – significant but not large – remains, but has begun to be bridged by the introduction of some free provision for four- and five-year-olds.

The situation pre-1997 in England and Scotland was very different. As in Sweden, compulsory schooling was free. But, unlike in Sweden, most parents were expected to pay the full costs of other services. The few exceptions included school-based early education for three- and four-year-olds where it was available, which unlike in Sweden was free;'children in need', whose'daycare' places were paid for by social services departments; and parents benefiting from the 'childcare disregard'. The difference between the UK and Sweden, which is significant and large, is basically unchanged post-1997, although rather more parents – though still not many – receive some fee subsidy through Childcare Tax Credit (CCTC). The Anglo-Scottish funding system consists of a mixture of supply subsidy (mainly for early education and compulsory schooling), demand subsidy (CCTC) and parental fees, backed up by various funding streams intended for 'pump priming', training and other activities intended to support market and workforce development. The result, as we have seen, is that Swedish parents pay higher taxes but lower fees than English and Scottish parents.

Second, regulation. We have already noted differences in the three countries' regulatory regimes with respect to levels of centralisation and decentralisation, and the extent of national prescription as opposed to local responsibility and interpretation. The extent of integration also varies. Since 1996, the three services that are the focus of this book have been subject in Sweden to a common curricular approach. This common approach, covering children from one to 16 years of age in pre-schools and schools (including school-age childcare), is articulated in two curriculum documents, one for pre-schools and the other for pre-school classes, schools and school-age childcare services. Both are the direct result of departmental integration, since prior to this there was a curriculum only for schools.

The documents are very similar. Both are short, cover a broad area and follow a common structure, starting with a discussion of fundamental values and tasks of the pre-school/school, and then setting out goals and guidelines (starting with norms and values). Both offer frameworks, leaving much to the interpretation of local authorities, institutions and practitioners. There are no national standards or child assessment systems until children reach age 11. There is a national agency – National Agency for Education – responsible for supervision of the full range of services within education, but it has employed a very informal style of inspection, which emphasises discussion.

England, by contrast, has three curricular or practice frameworks, one for children under three years, another for children aged from three to five years and the third for older children. These take very different forms, but are all detailed and specific. In England, they are combined with a system for assessing children from five years upwards, which again takes a different form for younger and older children: Foundation Stage profiling for five-year-olds, and Standard Assessment Tests currently from seven years upwards but in future for 11- and 15-year-olds as seven-year-olds are to be assessed using less formal methods. One agency inspects all childcare services and schools on a regular and formal basis, but in doing so works with a variety of regulations: integration is, again, partial.

Scotland has three curricular guidelines, one for three- to five-year-olds, one for five- to 14-year-olds and one for 14- to 16-year-olds. So far, there is nothing for children under three years, though such a curriculum is currently being prepared. These guidelines are, however, far less prescriptive than their English counterparts. Nor is there any centralised system of child assessment. The inspection of childcare and education remains split between welfare and education inspectorates, although joint inspections are planned for some services. The regulatory regime in Scotland, therefore, while closer to England's than to Sweden's, differs from England's in some significant respects.

The extent and nature of integration: principles

Moving services from welfare into education involves more than simply a change in departmental responsibility or a change of structures, whether through merging or through bringing them into new relationships. It also involves moving from one regime or environment of government to another, each with its distinctive mindsets, values, cultures and traditions – in this case from a 'welfare' to an 'education' rationality. An important dimension of integration, therefore, is what happens to the principles that are produced by the values, cultures and traditions of different systems and departments. Does transfer of responsibility lead to common policy principles being applied to all services gathered into the same department, whether through the transferred services adopting the principles of their new department or through the adoption of new shared principles by all concerned?

In Sweden, the transfer to education has led to the introduction of some key principles of the education system into services previously located in welfare. Within a short period, they have become 'educationalised' in important ways. In particular, new principles of access, funding and regulation have been introduced.

Previously, in welfare, access to early childhood and school-age childcare services had been conditional: entitlement to a place was restricted to children meeting certain need criteria, including having parents in employment or studying full-time, or children with special needs. Between 2001 and 2002, the entitlement became unconditional and therefore universal. This did not, in practice, involve a widespread change, since most Swedish parents are employed; the right of access was extended in effect to children with parents on parental leave or who are unemployed, and for these children the entitlement is limited to part-time hours. However, the new entitlement has broken the link between access and need, in particular parental employment, putting these services on the same footing as schools.

A change of perspective is under way here. Policy in Sweden is switching to the importance of all children (or at least those from 12 months or so of age) going to pre-school rather than reserving admission to children meeting required conditions. This means working to draw in the relatively small proportion of children whose parents choose not to send them to pre-schools, including children whose parents are not employed. A senior civil servant felt that one reason why 1996 was the right time for transferring pre-schools to education was that the traditions and values of education might make it better at the task of including all children.

The introduction of a period of free attendance at pre-schools from 2003 has inserted another educational principle into former welfare services, albeit partially because free attendance has not yet been extended universally to all children attending. At the same time, though, national government has offered funding to local authorities to enable them to apply a nationally determined maximum parental fee for services, to which parents still need to make a financial contribution. These funding reforms have been presented by the Swedish government as explicitly bringing pre-schools more closely into line with the education principles 'underlying all schools'.

We have already referred to new curricular frameworks under construction. But the introduction of a pre-school curriculum and the inclusion of free-time services within the curriculum of the school can also be seen as inserting the principles of the education system into services previously in the welfare system. Not only is a curriculum an educational concept and practice, but the form of the new pre-school curriculum, modelled on the school curriculum, makes it clear that an education system approach has been deliberately extended to include pre-schools and the whole age range of children attending them, not just those over three years of age. While there are significant differences between the pre-school and school documents, there are also significant similarities, not least in the formulation of values. Both documents, for example, begin by declaring that democracy forms the basis for pre-schools/schools and go on to state that everyone working in the pre-school/school should promote 'respect for the individual value of each person as well as respect for our shared environment'. The main difference between the two curricula is that the compulsory school curriculum is more subject-oriented than that of the pre-school, containing references, for example, to the acquisition of other languages and of domestic science.

To turn to England and Scotland, there is much less evidence of services formerly in the welfare system – 'childcare' – adopting education principles. Entitlement to services, beyond compulsory schooling, has been introduced, but only in the most limited way: part-time early education for three- and four-year-olds. The funding of services still follows very different principles: free for early education and compulsory schooling, parental fees (with limited subsidy to lower-income families) for other services. In England, the Foundation Stage and the National Curriculum adopt very different approaches. In Scotland, the pre-school curriculum is linked to the 5-14 guidelines through the use of key strands, but its focus on play is markedly different from the learning outcomes of those guidelines.

Relations with other services and policies for children

Much policy development in England and Scotland since 1997 has been concerned with finding new and more effective ways to address a range of government-targeted social problems. Central to this has been the promotion of improved working between agencies and the joining up of services so that they work together on agreed objectives and targets. Priority has been attached to breaking down old boundaries and adopting a cross-sectoral and cross-agency approach, which is focused on these common ends. The New Labour modernisation agenda calls for more responsive and 'joined-up' approaches, not hampered by administrative or bureaucratic rigidities.

In Scotland, the approach is typified by the report *For Scotland's children,* which promotes the creation of a single unitary children's service. Similarly, in England, the joined-up agenda links to the government's overarching strategy for children and young people with its framework of outcomes for children and young people applicable across government, and most recently with the establishment of a Minister and Directorate for Children, Young People and Families whose remit covers a wide range of diverse services. The theme of closer working relations and more 'joined up' approaches also runs through the English Green Paper, *Every child matters* (DfES, 2003a), though the frequent but undefined use of the word 'integration' can give a misleading impression of what is envisaged: integration, in terms of merging, is largely restricted to departmental reorganisation.

Many initiatives have been taken, or are planned, which include childcare and/or schools as part of a wider, joined-up approach to addressing particular issues. New agencies and partnerships, such as Sure Start programmes or the proposed Children's Trusts, bring together a wide range of services and staff to deliver specific objectives. New configurations of services, such as New Community Schools or Children's Centres, bring together a range of resources and occupational groups, with the rationale again of providing a more effective means of achieving policy aims. Some new types of worker may emerge in response to these new agencies and services. A recent report on the future of social care (the generic term used in England and Scotland to refer to work involving child protection and welfare) envisages a transformation in the workforce:

> The continued existence of separate professions working closely with the same service groups presents a major barrier to delivering more user focused services. [It is argued] that a major realignment of professional boundaries will be required in future and ultimately the creation of new professions. For example, a new profession combining youth and community work, social work, adolescent mental health services and career services could emerge to provide more holistic services for young people.... The seeds of these new professions have already been planted, through joint courses in nursing and social work and in new agencies like Connexions. They are being driven partly by the recognition that models of service provision based on society as it was in the 1940s – where the concept of teenager did not exist and where there were much shorter periods of retirement – are no longer appropriate. (Kendall and Harker, 2002, pp 11-12)

What is so far missing is any suggestion of new occupations that might span education, childcare and social care, or indeed any reform of the traditional schoolteacher. Most structural reforms of occupations are, so far, being mooted mainly within the welfare/social care sector.

The high priority attached to cross-agency work and joined-up services targeted at social problems, or indeed to social problems themselves – such as poverty and social exclusion – is not really apparent in Sweden at national or local level. Whereas it is difficult to see how we could have conducted our study in England and Scotland without being made constantly aware, from the start, of this wider policy context and the high priority attached to reducing poverty and social exclusion, nothing similar emerged during our time in Sweden. This is not to say there are no inter-agency or cross-service developments, nor is it to suggest that Sweden has no social problems. It is just to point out that such topics had no saliency in our interviews or in the documents we read.

It would be wrong, however, to conclude that early childhood education and care, schools and school-age childcare in Sweden exist in isolation, separated from other services or policies. As we have seen, there is a tradition of Swedish schools assuming a welfare role, and many schools have substantial input from nurses and social workers/counsellors. But the strongest example of 'joined-up' working is public support for employed parents: leave and services are both well-developed and closely connected in a way that they are not in the UK. Sweden recognised early on that such policies have a central place in family support in a post-industrial economy. By contrast, the English Green Paper, *Every child matters*, has a chapter devoted to 'Supporting parents and carers' that makes no reference to parental employment.

What's going on?

Our starting point was departmental integration of responsibility for early childhood services, compulsory schooling and school-age childcare services, a restructuring that occurred in three countries at around the same time. Having looked at the larger policy picture, we can see that this particular reform is part of different processes going on in our three countries. It has different significance and meanings in England, Scotland and Sweden.

In Sweden, it has been an integral part of a reform process underpinned by a new importance attached to lifelong learning and new understandings of the child, learning and knowledge. The reform process has been universal in scope and pedagogical in nature. The intention is to create an integrated and universal educational system spanning the whole of childhood and including pre-schools, compulsory schooling and free-time care services. This system is based on common structures, principles and concepts, including a common approach to children, learning and care.

In England and Scotland, departmental integration of responsibility for these services has been a more marginal part of a reform process concerned primarily to produce more effective interventions against a cluster of linked social and economic problems. The intention has been to join up existing agencies and services, sometimes creating new ones, sometimes enabling more collaborative working, to provide a more coherent and effective response to these problems. The reform process has been mainly targeted and welfarist in nature.

We need to unpack this highly concentrated conclusion. In mid-1990s Sweden, sustained public investment had ensured that employed or studying parents needing childcare could access a publicly funded service. It would be wrong to say that childcare was no longer important – it has to be in a society where so many parents are employed – but it was no longer a major policy issue. The country certainly was facing some new and challenging situations, including a recession bringing unparalleled levels of unemployment and some welfare cutbacks, and a recent increase in the minority ethnic population. However, levels of poverty and inequality had not reached crisis levels. Crisis was avoided by well-established policies to support parental employment and to redistribute income, both of which sprang from a welfare regime based on egalitarian principles and universal coverage.

In Sweden, the absence of widespread chronic social problems created space for an integration process focused on learning and education. But this is far from the whole story. There were many other influences favouring this outcome. There is a long-standing history of public discussion about the relationship between education and childcare. Services in the welfare system, especially pre-schools, have long been recognised to combine care and learning, welfare and education. A shift in emphasis to foreground learning, rather than a basic reconceptualisation, was all that was required.

The concept of pedagogy, applied to these services, is important here. It conveys the idea that care and learning are interrelated and inseparable, an idea expressed in the new pre-school curriculum, according to which the "pre-school should provide children with good pedagogical activities where care, nurturing and learning together from a coherent whole" (Swedish Ministry of Education and Science, 1998, p 8). Pedagogy is therefore an integrative concept, which starts from an assumption of wholeness rather than from the need to join up distinct domains such as care, education and health.

The process of integration – of services and policy principles – took place within a rather favourable climate: it is as if, after much foretelling, the time for integration in education had come, not only because the welfare mission (childcare) had been achieved but because a new educational challenge facing society had been recognised. This climate also included a discourse about the meaning of childhood, knowledge and learning in a post-industrial and knowledge society, a discourse that provides a rationale for a new and education-focused relationship between the three services. The Prime Minister at the time of integration, Göran Persson, himself a former education minister, declared in 1996: "Sweden must become a nation of knowledge, requiring improvements across the whole education system from pre-schools to universities and a lifelong learning perspective" (Lenz Taguchi and Munkammer, 2003).

Lifelong learning became a high policy priority in the 1990s, the Swedish Ministry of Education and Science (2000) noting that "the role of the pre-school in the information society and lifelong learning becomes very clear". The pre-school curriculum states that pre-schooling is the first step in a lifelong learning process. But the concept of lifelong learning, and arguments about its importance for future success, have also been taken on board by many parents, contributing to a near universal demand for early childhood services – now from all social classes – and an expectation that they will provide not only care but also opportunities for learning:

> [In Sweden] during the 1990s, early childhood education and care became the first choice for most working and studying parents.... Enrolling children from age one in full-day pre-schools has become generally acceptable. What was once viewed as either a privilege of the wealthy for a few hours a day or an institution for needy children and single mothers has become, after 70 years of political vision and policy-making, an unquestionable right of children and families. Furthermore, parents now expect *a holistic pedagogy that includes health care, nurturing and education* for their pre-schoolers.... [A]cceptance of full-day pre-schooling and schooling has complemented the idea of lifelong learning and the understanding of education as encompassing far more than imparting basic skills such as reading, writing and mathematics. (Lenz Taguchi and Munkammar 2003, p 27; emphasis added)

Lifelong learning relates to a wider discussion about knowledge and learning as well as about children and childhood. Note in the above quotation not only the significance of lifelong learning, but also the reference to an 'understanding of education as encompassing far more than imparting basic skills such as reading, writing and mathematics'. What has been emerging from this wider discussion is a view of the child, of knowledge and of learning that is increasingly widely held and that is supportive of the transfer of services from welfare to education. It is supportive because it foregrounds an understanding of the child as an active learner from birth, which entails the child seeking to construct knowledge and make meaning of the world around it, and also because it opens up to the possibility of a new and equal relationship between early childhood education and care, schools and school-age childcare based on new and shared understandings rather than a takeover by schools and a narrowly didactic view of education.

This last point is a prominent feature of the Swedish integration process: the idea that integration involves *vertical* (pre-school/school) relationships as well as *horizontal* (care/education) relationships. Moreover, integration involving vertical relationships should not be centred on compulsory schooling and its traditions but, on the contrary, should treat pre-schools as equal partners with an important contribution to make to the whole field of education:

> State directives have always stressed coordination and cooperation between pre-school and compulsory schooling. The idea has been to make the transition between the two as smooth as possible for the children, by bringing the two pedagogies closer together. With the extension of the holistic view of the child into schooling, children enjoy continuity and a sense of self-assurance in the new learning institution. The holistic approach puts equal emphasis on all aspects of the child's development – the emotional, social and physical (i.e. motor abilities) as well as cognitive. The different learning

environments and cultures were expected to complement rather than contradict each other during the first years of schooling. The rhetorical logic was, thus, that pre-schooling was to influence schooling (in the early years), rather than make children start compulsory schooling earlier. (Lenz Taguchi and Munkammar 2003, pp 12-13)

Discussion in Sweden of vertical integration, involving relations between pre-schools and schools, has also gone beyond rhetoric. These relations have been theorised by two Swedish researchers in an influential paper prepared in 1994 for a government commission, the name of whose report – *The base for lifelong learning: A school ready for children* (*Grunden för livslångt larande: En barnmogen skola*) – reflects both the importance attached to lifelong learning from birth and the idea that compulsory school may need to change. The paper provides a critical analysis of the different cultures of the pre-school and school and of the "possibilities and risks involved in an integration of the two educational forms". From this analysis, it goes on to offer "a vision of a possible meeting place between the pre-school and school". It provides a unique and powerful aid to thinking about the integration of pre-schools within the education system – what the deep-seated obstacles are, how they might be overcome, how it might look.

The paper – titled *Pre-school and school – Two different traditions and a vision of an encounter* (*Förskola och skola – om två skilda traditioner och om visionem om en mötesplats*) (Dahlberg and Lenz Taguchi, 1994) – begins by identifying different pedagogical traditions in pre-school and school, each produced by a different social construction of the child: "the analysis shows that the view of the child which we call the child as nature is, for the most part, embodied in the pre-school, while the child as producer of culture and knowledge is, for the most part, embodied in the school". These different constructions have had "direct consequences on the content and working methods of pedagogical activity, and in that way affected the view of the child's learning and knowledge-building". The paper goes on to suggest an alternative construction of the child, namely, as a constructor of culture and knowledge – which could "create a meeting place" where both the pre-school teachers and the primary school teachers are given the possibility to develop their pedagogical practices:

> We do not wish to present a new pedagogical method or model, but a vision of a possible meeting place. This vision can be seen as a provisional, holistic picture of the educational institutions we need in a quickly changing society. The vision deals with a way of relating and a working process in relation to the child's creation of knowledge and everyday reality which is based upon continual discussions and common values which one wants to permeate the child's upbringing and education. This way of relating starts from the view of the child as a competent and capable child, a rich child, who participates in the creation of themselves and their knowledge – the child as a constructor of culture and knowledge. In this pedagogical approach,

> this way of relating is characterised by a researching, reflective and analytical approach at different levels. (Dahlberg and Lenz Taguchi, 1994)

It is important to emphasise that the discussion of vertical integration – between pre-school and school – includes the horizontal integration of education and care at all levels or, in the terms we have described earlier, its scope is that of a holistic pedagogy. Pre-school and school should be moving to new, shared positions on learning rather than confronting children with two different approaches. But they should also provide other continuity for children – for example, a shared concern with care and security, as expressed by the 'red thread' metaphor.

To sum up, the transfer of responsibility for services from welfare to education in Sweden can be seen as part of a larger and long-term integrative process, in which locating departmental responsibility for pedagogical services within education was, if not inevitable, then certainly not surprising. As childcare needs were met, attention was turned to other aspects of the work of 'integrated' pre-schools, in particular learning; responsibility for schools was devolved to local authorities, bringing all three services into their remit and stimulating local departmental integration; school-age childcare was increasingly integrated with schools; departmental responsibility was integrated at a national level; pre-schools and free-time services have been included in the curricular regime, universal entitlement has been extended from schools to pre-schools and some free pre-school provision has been introduced; workforce training is being integrated, with a new qualification for a new kind of teacher.

This broad, integrative, education-based process has met no major opposition, political, professional or otherwise: one trade union, for example, already covers most workers in the different professions involved. The services transferred from welfare 'fit' easily into education: forming part of a Nordic welfare regime, they already had much in common with educational principles, in particular a recognition that they are a public good, extensive (if not quite universal) entitlement, a professionalised workforce and large-scale (if not exclusive) public funding. We have already noted that neither shortage of 'childcare' nor poverty was a major issue, which might otherwise have distracted attention.

In Sweden, therefore, we see strong continuities before and after 1996. The same is true of England and Scotland, although in very different ways. Before and after 1997, policy evinces a view of childcare as a mainly private commodity, limited entitlement for parents and children, a strong tendency to target needy populations, a mainly non-professionalised workforce and limited public funding. In England and Scotland, too, the situation of services was very different from that in Sweden at the time responsibility was transferred. Instead of an already integrated and rather strong early childhood service, there was a plethora of services divided between welfare and education in a weak system – weak because the early age at which children start school truncates the system, because of slow development and sustained under-investment, and because of the fragmentation of services, which creates different interest groups. Services within the welfare system were mainly provided privately, often for profit, while services in the education system were mainly provided publicly. The main occupational groups had very different training, pay and other conditions – for example, access to occupational pensions. In a liberal welfare regime, inclined to targeted public provision and otherwise requiring the operation of private responsibility, there was a gulf between the principles underpinning 'childcare' and 'education' services. There was no integrative concept in common use, such as pedagogy: while some experts might argue that childcare and education were inseparable, 'childcare' was usually discussed as a separate issue by politicians, the media and the public at large. One reason it was discussed in this way was the relatively low levels of childcare provision for working parents: unlike in Sweden, childcare was far from being a need that had been met.

The UK Labour government came to power with a set of problems in its domestic policy sights: reducing poverty and social exclusion; reducing worklessness; raising educational attainments; improving economic productivity and competitiveness. While 'lifelong learning' and the 'knowledge society' appear in government documents, they take second place to these seemingly more pressing issues. While 'childcare' might have an educational element, as most policy documents acknowledge, it has been viewed by many sections of government, including the Treasury, as primarily a means to reduce poverty and worklessness by enabling parents to participate in the labour market.

'Childcare', therefore, retains a separate identity in the eyes of many people. It is regarded as a kind of rootless or free-floating service that contributes to meeting a range of policy ends and tackling many problem areas. Viewed from this perspective, it is no more closely connected to education than many other policy areas; there is, therefore, no reason to privilege the childcare relationship with education at the expense of any other policy relationship. Many departments have an interest in childcare, but most have little awareness of, or particular interest in, education or its relation to care: complex and contentious issues of theory and practice in work with children are avoided by references to 'quality' and 'child development', which suggest that technical solutions are readily available for such issues and that further discussion is not required.

This perception of 'childcare' as distinct and different pervades government policy and is expressed in the language used. Key policy documents include *Meeting the* **Childcare** *challenge*, which sets out a *National* **Childcare** *Strategy* and an *interdepartmental* **childcare** *review*. A further review of *childcare* policies, announced by the Chancellor of the Exchequer, reports in 2004. Funding strategies have including the *Childcare* Tax Credit and promoting 'the business case for various forms of *childcare* assistance'. Policy makers refer to *childcare* services, *childcare* providers and the *childcare* workforce. In this context, it is possible for a leading practitioner magazine to ask whether "education (is) being eclipsed by care in the Government's moves against poverty and social disadvantage" (Evans, 2003a, p 10).

The location of 'childcare' within government, therefore, is not inevitably in education. Indeed, from the perspective of government, in England at least, there has appeared to be a strong case for its administrative location to be where responsibility for employment resides. The employment interest, therefore, has acted throughout as a gravity field pulling childcare away from being fully integrated with education. With the movement of responsibility for employment out of education, the influences that brought childcare into education were no longer sufficient to prevent its being partly brought out again, to become the joint responsibility of education and employment departments.

This perception of childcare and a reluctance to integrate it with education needs to be seen as concomitant with a wider government strategy for undertaking its big economic and social projects. Problems are identified, objectives set, then agencies and services are brought into play to achieve the objectives – often through the mediation of new agencies or partnerships. This 'joined-up' work involves a long menu of services and occupations beyond childcare and education: health, child welfare, family support and many others. Viewed against this vast backdrop, integrating childcare and education, merging them structurally and conceptually, is an irrelevance, even a distraction from the goals of getting more childcare places to support a raft of policies and outcome-focused work across a range of services. Childcare and early education are now treated as but a part of a wide range of services for children, now the responsibility of one minister but which do not, however, include 'mainstream schools and education policy' – although these also are governed by the need to meet the main policy agenda, using a variety of technical means.

Integrating services seems less relevant and effective, therefore, than finding ways for separate services to work more closely together, in different relationships and configurations for different purposes, or, where necessary, creating new services. For example, rather than the Swedish concept of the whole-day school, which aims at an integration of early education, compulsory education and free-time care, English extended schools will become bases for a number of different services, including school-age childcare. Similarly, in Scotland, the commitment to making every school an integrated community school by 2007 gives priority to the involvement of different agencies, such as health and social work, rather than to any restructuring of the school itself, although the National Debate on Education Action Plan does include provision for a pilot project on alternative structures to the school day.

Integration has also been affected by the existence of different views and traditions about education, which produce different understandings of learning and knowledge. In England, the Foundation Stage and the National Curriculum reflect such differences: one more child-centred and play-oriented, the other more subject-based and formal. While the Foundation Stage may act as a barrier to formal education being pushed further down into the earliest years of childhood, it has had little success in pushing its ethos up into compulsory schooling, where one consequence of recent reforms, with their emphasis on choice and markets, has been a populist and 'reinvigorated traditionalism' (Whitty et al, 1998, p 13). In the traditional model, the child is understood as a reproducer of knowledge, a being who starts life as an empty vessel and who needs to be made 'ready to learn' and 'ready for school' where she can be filled with socially sanctioned knowledge, skills and values (Dahlberg et al, 1999, pp 44-5).

Rather than a search for a new, shared understanding of knowledge and learning related to a common social construction of the child, there appears to be increasing tension between early years and compulsory education, a tension recognised and described by several informants. No vision of a new meeting place is apparent, nor has any critical analysis of the subject – the relationship between pre-school and compulsory school – been commissioned. Evidence is endlessly sought about the effectiveness of different technologies and practices, but there is little interest in more conceptual issues and critical analysis.

Highlighting the difference

We have argued that the transfer of responsibility for a range of so-called childcare services from welfare into education was a central part of an ongoing and wide-ranging educational reform in Sweden, but a more peripheral part of a programme to tackle a range of social and economic problems in England and Scotland. In Sweden, 'childcare' was seen as inseparable from learning; in England and Scotland, 'childcare' was a means to many ends. This distinction can be highlighted if we cite the example of a fourth country that has transferred all pre-school services to education.

New Zealand took this step in 1986. The relevance to our discussion resides in its many similarities with England and Scotland, and dissimilarities with Sweden – except for the educational focus of its reform process. New Zealand, like the UK, has gone through a period of strong neo-liberal experimentation, which brought with it high levels of child poverty (Blaiklock et al, 2002): "only in New Zealand, where neoliberal policies were even more radical and the egalitarian inheritance more pronounced, did inequality grow faster [than Britain]" (Gray, 1998, p 32). Like England and Scotland, New Zealand's early childhood services were diverse, mainly privately provided and not so developed as Sweden's. They included childcare centres (nurseries), kindergartens providing part-time provision for three- and four-year-olds, play centres (playgroups), pre-school classes attached to primary schools, various services specifically for Maori and other minority ethnic groups, and family daycarers. As in England and Scotland, government responsibility for these pre-school services, pre-transfer, was split between the departments of education (kindergartens) and welfare (other services).

But the transfer of departmental responsibility for all services to education has, unlike in England and Scotland but like in Sweden, clearly been part of an education-focused reform process. This is evident from three features. First, a national early childhood curriculum, *Te Whaariki*, covering all services and all pre-school children, has been adopted. Meade and Podmore (2001) attach great importance to the role of this framework in the integration process:

> It remains exceedingly rare for countries to give official recognition to a curriculum for infants and toddlers, and for countries to assume that an early childhood curriculum will be implemented with similar effectiveness in childcare centres and kindergartens. In New Zealand, the development and implementation of *Te Whaariki* as the national curriculum for children from birth to (at least) 5 years, appears to have been a critical success factor. The type of curriculum has contributed to *the pedagogical integration of care and education*, and to the avoidance of 'educationalisation' or a top-down approach to the learning and teaching of infants and young children. It is not a subject-based curriculum. Rather, it reflects the wider role of early childhood education: it focuses on empowering all involved to foster children's well-being and sense of belonging so that children become confident and competent communicators and learners. (Meade and Podmore, 2001, p 47; emphasis added)

Second, a single funding framework has been established, with a common subsidy formula covering all services, based on the number of child hours of attendance, with an extra payment for children aged under two years. However, even with the subsidy, not all types of services can be offered free of charge, and a fee subsidy (paid by the welfare ministry) is available to low-income families using services defined as providing 'childcare'. Thus, the funding system, as in our three countries, is not yet fully integrated: "the continuation of this [fee] subsidy only for families using childcare services through the last decade has the effect of continuing to separate education and care, albeit it in a limited way" (Meade and Podmore, 2001, p 43). The common subsidy formula, applied to all services, is part of an overall policy aim to treat all services equitably; the continuation of fee subsidy to some services goes against that attempt to bring all services within a common system of principles and values. Funding therefore demonstrates the aspiration of integration and the constraints on attaining this aspiration.

Third, steps have been taken to integrate the workforce, based on a new training introduced in 1987 leading to a new teaching qualification – Diploma in Education (early childhood teaching) – which has become regarded as a 'benchmark' early childhood qualification for staff working in different settings for children from birth to five years. The 2002 Strategic Plan for Early Childhood Education (New Zealand Ministry of Education, 2002) proposes that by 2012 all staff in 'teacher-led services' (which include childcare centres and kindergartens) will be required to have this qualification.

New Zealand, however, has not addressed the relationship between early childhood services and compulsory schooling, even to the limited extent of introducing, as in England and Scotland, a curriculum spanning the short transition period between pre-school and school (though the extension of *Te Whaariki* to the first year of compulsory schooling is under discussion). Rather, the focus is on the division between early childhood and compulsory schooling, and how to protect the former from the latter. Traditionally, in New Zealand:

> ... the values of early childhood education are not synonymous with those of school systems. Early childhood education has a history ... of a strong emphasis being placed on the nature of children and on the processes of learning. Conversely, educational curricula and testing in the school system have tended towards performance-based achievement models where the emphasis is on products of learning. These differences, and associated theories of learning and development, underpin *concerns about the possible escalation of 'educationalisation' of early childhood* through placing childcare services within the administrative auspices of education. (Meade and Podmore, 2001, p 47; emphasis added)

New Zealand provides us with an example from the English-speaking world of a country that is seeking to integrate all early childhood education and care services not only within the education system but with a strong emphasis on learning. Despite strong similarities in conditions, New Zealand has followed a markedly different path from England and Scotland. But only Sweden, having already achieved this horizontal integration between care and education in the years before compulsory schooling, is taking the next step: attempting to foster a strong, equal and integrated vertical relationship between early childhood services and compulsory schooling, drawing on a pedagogical tradition and based on new, shared understandings and practices.

SEVEN

Endnotes

The starting point for this study was three countries each taking the same step, moving responsibility in national government for a group of services for children from one department, namely, welfare, to another, namely, education. Yet, despite this initial similarity, what has proved more striking is the differences between the countries, in the measures taken before and after this act of transfer and in the meaning of the act itself. We have found differences in the structuring of services and the workforce, in the principles of provision, and in underlying concepts and understandings. Transfer in one case was an important step in a long-term process of educational reform. In the other cases it was a subsidiary measure in a broader process of creating more 'childcare' services and better coordinated relations between disparate services.

The cross-national differences we have documented are important in their own right, irrespective of what they mean for children. For they show the continuing influence of the nation state even at a time of increasing global capital flows and economic competition. The nation state may have been 'hollowed out' in some respects, losing power over important areas, especially economic. But our cases show that it remains strong in determining social arrangements. Tradition, culture and values still coalesce to create different responses to similar developments, in our cases including the increased policy importance of maternal employment and children's education. Herein lies the importance of the concept of welfare regime. This combination of typical ways of thinking, acting and allocating responsibility has provided one way of explaining differences between our countries as well as continuities within nations through periods of change.

What seems clear is that the Nordic welfare regime, as practised in Sweden, has worked rather well, at least in the pedagogic and educational areas we have studied, and at least in comparison with the liberal welfare regime exemplified by England and Scotland. Despite having to weather a harsh recession, Sweden has kept poverty and inequality far lower; a strong system of parental leave entitlements has been put in place; and accessible and affordable 'childcare' services have been built up to the point where they can now be offered as a universal right. (We place 'childcare' in inverted commas throughout this chapter as a constant reminder that it is a contested concept, especially in the context of a study that has raised the possibility of alternative ways of thinking about and giving effect to the relationship between care and education.)

Moreover, affordable services are combined with a professionalised workforce, better paid and trained than the workforce in comparable services in Britain. A question posed by this study and elsewhere (Moss and Cameron, 2002), is whether liberal welfare regimes, with their emphasis on private responsibility for 'care' services and their tendency to targeted 'demand' subsidies – for example, tax credits – can undertake the major revaluation and reform of the workforce that Sweden has achieved; or whether reliance on parental fees to fund services, mediated only by modest fee subsidy, and on 'for-profit' providers to deliver them will contribute not only to the maintenance of the status quo – for who can or will, in these circumstances, foot the bill to reform the conditions of the workforce? – but also to an increasing crisis of care as poorly paid care work is increasingly unable to recruit and retain its workforce.

The Nordic welfare state comes with a high price tag, mostly met by government. Taxes are high in Sweden. But this simple statement has too often served to divert attention from a more complex reality and contributed to an ill-informed dismissal (by many in English-speaking countries) of Nordic welfare states. Taxes may be lower in England and Scotland, but 'childcare' fees paid by parents are far higher and leave benefits far less generous, while poverty and inequality are abundant and abiding. In considering welfare regimes, the big spending picture needs to be considered. How much is paid *in toto* for benefits and services through public taxes but also by employers and individuals? What are the returns on this total expenditure? And how are costs and returns distributed?

Welfare regimes are important. They prove to be a useful explanatory tool, casting some light, for example, on the continuities in Britain's policy towards 'childcare' before and after 1997. 'New' Labour made 'childcare' a central plank of its economic and social project, a significant change of course. Yet the plank was recognisable, larger certainly than before, but similar in shape and material to smaller planks in earlier projects: it was cut from the same tree.

But, their importance having been acknowledged, welfare regimes should not be treated as inevitable and unchanging, nor are they entirely unmixed. Signs of a liberal regime can be detected in Sweden, including, for example, some moves to a more marketised approach to early years services with encouragement for private providers (who are, nevertheless subsidised to the same extent as public services); while the English and Scottish governments, though their main measures have been strongly targeted towards socially disadvantaged groups, have also adopted a rhetoric of universalism (DfES, 2003a).

Moreover, some analysts have suggested that recent changes in some liberal welfare states, such as the UK and Canada, suggest the emergence of a variant regime, 'the social investment state' (Dobrowolsky, 2002; Sevenhuijsen, 2002; Fawcett et al, 2003; Lister, 2003). This regime foregrounds the importance of the citizen being self-sufficient and productive through paid work, and the role of social expenditure in providing investment to sustain the nation's competitiveness in a global economy: expenditure on children's care and education is viewed as such an investment in the future. Lister (2003) identifies a number of key features of the social investment state: investment in social and human capital; children prioritised as future citizens and workers; redistribution of opportunities to promote social inclusion rather than of income to promote equality; adaptation of individuals and society to enhance global competitiveness; and integration of economic and social policy with the latter still the 'handmaiden' of the former. To the extent that the Swedish reforms have also been seen, in part at least, as a means to securing Sweden's place in a future global economy – for example, in the context of lifelong learning – there are some points in common, although these are outnumbered by the differences in values, principles and practices that underpin fundamentally different welfare regimes.

What will prove interesting to watch over future years is whether devolved Scotland decides to move away from England's liberal welfare orientation towards a more Nordic regime. Our study has shown many basic similarities between England and Scotland. Yet there are enough signs of difference, in both the language and practice of current policy, to suggest the potential for increasing divergence in the future. Scotland has shared with Sweden a greater propensity to discuss the issues involved, initiating, for example, a National Debate on Education addressing questions about why and how children learn and signalling a continuing commitment to public, comprehensive education. It is unlikely that any divergence would be formally announced and implemented by a Scottish Executive, and more likely that it might involve a gradual accretion of changes leading to an increasingly hybrid welfare regime. There are, too, major constraints anchoring Scotland to an English-type welfare regime, including the retention of important powers – in particular around the economy and employment – by the UK government, as well as the strengthened role of HM Treasury across the whole spectrum of domestic social policy. A major shift in welfare regime presumes not only substantial tax-raising powers but freedom to move, for example, from a tax-embedded system of demand subsidy (tax credits) to a tax-based system of supply subsidy and, more generally, from a targeted to a universal approach in public support for services.

Nor are the constituent parts of welfare regimes immutable. The transfer of departmental responsibility for early years and school-age 'childcare' services in Sweden, and the subsequent changes we have described, have decisively moved these services out of welfare and into education. Education might be considered a quite different type of regime from welfare, with a number of important principles and practices common across countries (not least the principles of universal entitlement and tax-based public funding). The gap in principles and provision between education and welfare varies between countries with, as we have shown, closer correspondence between education and welfare in Sweden than in England and Scotland.

While 'childcare' may continue to figure in cross-national comparisons of welfare regimes, such analyses will have to recognise that 'childcare' can be educationalised. This entails structural questions about where 'childcare' services are administratively located and how they are organised, but it also raises more conceptual questions. In such cases of educationalisation, does the concept of 'childcare services' retain meaning as a distinct field of policy and provision, or should the 'childcare' function be treated as a facet of education? Should services that may provide 'childcare' as one of their purposes be understood and treated as if they were substitutes for maternal care (as they are in much welfare state analysis) or, like schools, as institutions qualitatively different from the home, providing quite different relationships, possibilities and practices? The Swedish reform points to one possible future, in which the dualistic discussion and provision of 'childcare' and 'education' has been finally superseded by a more unified discourse of 'education in its broadest sense', a 'pedagogical' view of education, expressed in the emergence of a reformed and broadened education system, providing services from birth through to adulthood. Put another way, have the Swedes managed to get 'beyond childcare', treating parental needs for 'childcare' as a necessary, integral but subsidiary purpose of pre-schools and schools?

What this preamble suggests, and our study highlights, is the choices that governments face in making provision for children and young people. Underlying particular policy choices – the type of services to provide, how to provide, fund, regulate and staff them – are large questions. To look at the big national picture, it is necessary to ask: how well does the current welfare regime work? What direction should the welfare regime take? What relationship should welfare services have to education?

Our study has shown three countries producing different answers to the last question. The move of certain services into the education system in Sweden is part of a wider move towards reshaping and rethinking the education system. Early years services, school-age 'childcare' and schools are now parts of that system – integration as merging across a range of key dimensions (such as access, curricula, staffing, management, funding) is in progress. But a condition of the success of these changing relations is, in principle at least, that changes should flow through the whole system. Integration, in theory, should not mean takeover through 'schoolification'; rather, all parts should come together in a new meeting place of shared understandings and practices. Pedagogy as a concept and lifelong learning as a national necessity provide rationales for this new relationship, as too, perhaps, does the condition of childhood today in Sweden. From the age of a year or so, most Swedish children enter some form of societally sanctioned and publicly funded institution, first (in most cases) the pre-school, then (in most cases) the whole-day school. In these conditions, the question of relationships between what have become near-universal institutions of childhood – pre-schools, schools and free-time services – becomes critical. These relationships have been discussed in the past, over many years, but the momentum for vertical and horizontal integration appears to have become unstoppable in the 1990s.

For the Swedes, the key issue is the relationship between these services (and between them and leave policies for parents). Other issues – for example, the relationship between these universal services and more targeted services such as child welfare – have been less prominent. For the English and the Scots, however, there have been other preoccupations: building up what they refer to as 'childcare' services to enable increased labour market participation of women, and constructing coalitions of services to create more effective technologies for tackling particular social problems, especially poverty and social exclusion. Especially in Scotland, the school has loomed large in these coalitions, with the distinctive and early policy developments of both the pilot programme of New Community Schools now being rolled out to all schools and the 2002 National Debate on Education.

But there has been little by way of radical moves to integrate schools with other services – more often, services are located within the school. The idea, for example, that a 'childcare worker' might manage a school, or that teacher training might merge with 'childcare' training, or indeed that school and school-age 'childcare' might merge into a 'whole-day' provision remain unthinkable for the moment or, indeed, the foreseeable future: yet all are common practice in Sweden. Curricula, at least in England, are at odds with each other, the Foundation Stage confronting the National Curriculum, while in Sweden they provide a shared framework for early years services, schools and school-age 'childcare'.

Just as the school remains conceptually and structurally distinct in so much Anglo-Scottish policy language and practice, so, too, does 'childcare'. It is, perhaps, not surprising that it figures so prominently and distinctly, given years of public disregard of the need for working parents to have access to services that recognise and support their employment: the absence of something so important understandably makes obtaining it something of a preoccupation. But the continuing distinctiveness of 'childcare' – whether in policy, the media or daily conversation – goes deeper. It reflects the absence of alternative, more integrative concepts, like pedagogy, which start from a holistic perspective rather than requiring one to be constructed from scattered pieces. And it reflects, too, a construction of the young child as a simple and dependent being, whose proper place is in the private sphere of home and maternal care, until offered up to start education at primary school. If mothers must work, then the child needs some approximation to care at home, by 'nursery nurses' or 'childminders' (or preferably by a family member), perhaps with some 'preparation for school and learning' added for part of the time (take, for example, the continuing policy premise that early learning should be confined to a few hours a day, with the limited understanding of early learning that this view conveys).

Different relationships bring different opportunities and risks, some of which we hinted at in Chapter One. Integration in Sweden holds out the prospect of new thinking and practice in the field of learning, a flow of ideas and methods through the extended system, a radical reciprocity in which, for example, pedagogical work in the pre-school might be taken up and adapted for use in secondary school, just as innovative work in secondary school might feed back into the pre-school. Conversely, the risk remains of the schoolification of part or all of the system, of schools not finding the new meeting place and, as powerful institutions, their traditional ways of education permeating the whole day school or the pre-school. The popularity of the school teaching option among the first intake of students in the new training system is just one indicator of how hard it may prove to move from hierarchical to equal relationships.

The dangers of schoolification are not confined to less powerful services within an education system. We should be aware, too, of the risk arising from a large integrated system that has the child for nearly 20 years of her life and for a substantial part of the day. The risk is that this redesigned institutionalisation of childhood creates conditions for more effectively governing the child, not only in terms of producing desired outcomes but also through creating a desired subject, for example the autonomous, flexible, entrepreneurial subject of neo-liberal economics (for further discussion of how early childhood services may be implicated in such processes of subjectification, see Fendler, 2001). Of course, some might welcome such effective production. We are, however, less sympathetic to this concept of public provision for children as producers of predetermined outcomes and as sites for governing the soul (Moss and Petrie, 2002), and suggest that increased integration needs to go hand in hand with increased opportunities and capabilities for critical thinking among practitioners, parents, policy makers and politicians.

More 'joined up' working across a wider range of services creates opportunities for more effective interventions to prevent or ameliorate a range of social problems. The New Community School or local Sure Start programme may, for example, be able to coordinate and deploy a range of professions and skills to better help individual children and their families. But a risk arises from expecting too much of services and professionals in addressing problems, in particular poverty and inequality, which have their origins in economic systems and welfare regimes. The balance between agency and structure can tilt too much towards agency and the naïve belief that poverty can be eliminated through the agency of poor people, 'empowered' by education and employment delivered through service intervention. In the face of a hundred years or more of service interventions intended to solve the problem of the poor, such beliefs betray an inadequate understanding of structural causes. This is not to argue against closer relations between services and occupations, but to suggest the limitations of 'joined-upness' and 'modernisation' – the limitations of services however well deployed.

Another risk arises if insufficient attention is paid to understanding the deep-seated systemic obstacles to 'joined-upness'. One concern is the intrinsic difficulty of bringing different systems (and those who work within them) into closer working relationships. Michael King (1997, p 26) has written about how "each [system] is closed to its external world in the sense that information from the world cannot penetrate the system in a direct manner ... [but] has to be reproduced in the system's own terms". In other words, each system sees the world through its own lens, and each system formulates problems in terms of its own agenda and perceived competence: direct communication between systems is always problematic, since "these systems are able to relate to one another only by attempting to impose their own self-generated evaluations and criteria for success upon the other" (King, 1997, p 205). The Swedish study of different traditions and cultures in pre-schools and schools referred to earlier (see Chapter Six) provides a good example of how, once recognised, these systemic differences can be analysed and worked on – the operative words being 'once recognised'.

A consequence of the reforms we have described is that the childhoods children live in the three countries are increasingly differentiated because of the growing significance of institutions in childhood and the widening gap in national policy, provision and practice concerning these institutions. To take one example, a five-year-old in Sweden will be nearing the end of her time in a pre-school, which she may well have attended since the age of 12 to 15 months. Most of her fellow five-year-olds from where she lives will attend the same pre-school. The staff in the pre-school will mostly be pre-school teachers (perhaps in 2005 also one or two of the first graduates from the new teacher training). The staff will enjoy considerable autonomy, with opportunities to develop their own pedagogical theories and practice within the broad remit of the national curriculum and its local interpretation. The next year, when six, she will go to school, where she may well be part of a 'whole-day school' group of six- to eight- or nine-year-olds, educated and cared for by a team of professional workers. A *rektor* – perhaps a pre-school teacher – will have overall responsibility for both the pre-school and the school.

At the other extreme, an English five-year-old will probably be at the end of her first reception year in primary school or starting her second year, coming up to or just past the border between Foundation Stage and National Curriculum. She will probably have been to an early years service prior to entering reception class, in fact very likely to more than one. But the exact course of this 'career' – how many placements, of what type, with whom – will depend on many factors, including where she lives, her parents' employment and their income. As a five-year-old at school, if her parents' employment does not coincide with school hours and holidays, she will need an additional 'childcare' arrangement, necessitating yet more different carers and a different environment. This will add to the number and variety of adults through whose hands she will have passed, including some or all out of nursery workers, playgroup workers, childminders, teachers and school-based assistants. The staff in her school class will be governed by national requirements, including a detailed curriculum and assessment regime, and the school itself will be subject, from time to time, to detailed scrutiny by a national inspectorate.

It seems to us that it is of the utmost importance to better understand these different environments and regimes in which children live their childhoods and which result from different policies, provisions and practices, and to do so from both adult and child perspectives. If we, as adults, require childhood to be institutionalised, then we need to ask questions about what type of childhood results, about both the opportunities and the risks. Answers to such questions provide material for a critical evaluation – not only in terms of consequences but also in terms of children's lives. Do our arrangements provide a good childhood? And this, of course, is an ethical and political question.

All three countries have been engaged in the implementation of major policy changes, whether involving moves to integration or the expansion of services and the promotion of more joined-up working. Our study therefore necessarily raises questions about the conditions needed to bring about such major changes, what in Britain at least has become termed 'the reform of public services'. In one respect at least, Sweden has had a clear advantage. Transfer of departmental responsibility and the other changes associated with it have occurred at a time when the services transferred have already been built up to provide near-universal cover. In England and Scotland, by contrast, much attention has been devoted to boosting the supply of provision, to the extent that in the case of 'childcare' this has become a (or in some cases the) major preoccupation.

This reflects a historical difference. The reforms we studied in Sweden are part of a steady process of development, going back to the 1960s, when the expansion of services began in response to growing maternal employment. But many of the issues involved, such as the relation between care and education and the role of the school, go back well before this time. While recent Swedish reforms have involved some major changes (notably the reform of training), they come with a widely understood history which has sensitised key players to the issues and the possibilities. The reforms in the 1990s have an evolutionary feel to them, not an inevitability but a probability. They have been eased by strong political and cultural continuities, and also by a strong democratic tradition that has left an important legacy of knowledge and understanding from a succession of commissions and studies. The recent Swedish reforms can be seen as part of a political and cultural process by which Swedish society has reflected upon itself and its children.

By contrast, reforming the relationship between services in England and Scotland has been treated in a less historical and more technical way. Change has been driven by a set of new policy imperatives, most notably to improve certain forms of educational attainment and to increase the numbers of 'childcare services'. As these are major government commitments, priority has been attached to showing quick results, forcing the relationship between care and education into, at best, second place and, at worst, no place at all. It has created an anomalous relationship to the past. Existing forms of 'childcare' and approaches to education – the historical legacy – were maintained and built on, so to that extent the past was influential. But there was no conscious historical perspective, no attempt to understand the origins of the legacy, to look at past experience or indeed discussions, no time or inclination to take stock. The tone was set by the first major government policy documents in England and Scotland, which set out a 'childcare strategy' rather than, for example, taking the form of broader and more considered green papers on the future development of, and the relationship between, early years services, school-age 'childcare' and education. Diagnosis of current inadequacies and prescriptions for future action were not complemented by reflections on past experience.

This is symptomatic of a certain absence of thought behind the post-1997 measures, in favour of action expressed in a constant flow of initiatives, targets and other demands from central government. Change, in short, has been strongly top-down (although a number of local authorities have been ahead of the game). In England and Scotland, central departments have sought to combine policy making and implementation, relying on overworked civil servants, often passing through rather rapidly, with no solid core of experienced, long-serving officials. A 'command and control' tendency has been exacerbated, in England, by the Treasury taking a great interest in affairs, pressing for more 'childcare', with little background or interest in the question of how care and education are related. HM Treasury also casts its influence over Scotland, through, for example, its control of public subsidies for 'childcare' services (Childcare Tax Credits), which are premised on private market provision, as well as initiatives such as Sure Start that cut across devolved areas of responsibility.

Change in Sweden has been driven, to a considerable extent, by local authorities in the context of a high degree of decentralisation, but has been complemented by central government decisions, including the transfer of responsibility for schools to local authorities, legislation giving entitlement to places, funding arrangements and training. Central government certainly played a more directive role in the 1970s, in the earlier stages of service development. But it has now relaxed its grip, accepting and welcoming local diversity, and trusting both local democracy and professional capabilities. By English and Scottish standards, Sweden may have a very uniform system of services, most young children, for example, attending municipal pre-schools. Yet by Swedish standards, English and Scottish services must conform to an extremely prescriptive system of centralised regulation. Which countries have greater diversity depends therefore on which dimensions of diversity are being considered.

The issue, perhaps, in Sweden is how the almost revolutionary change anticipated in education can be brought about in practice. How does one change strong institutions like schools, in particular the higher grades? (And given the influence of each level of education on the one below, the long-term response of the higher grades of schooling to the education reforms could well prove critical.) How does one create strong, equal and reciprocal relations? How does one put into practice the 'vision of a new meeting place' that recognises and respects the traditions and cultures of pre-schools and schools but also seeks to create new, shared understandings and practices? How is a new profession, open to new ideas and radical reciprocity, brought into being?

Such changes cannot be legislated to happen: no amount of government guidance will ensure compliance. But nor can they simply be left to take their own course. How such far-reaching change can best be fostered and realised remains unclear. We would, however, suggest four conditions. First, making time for thought. Unless change is understood simply as applying new rules from the top, then time for local discussion and reflection, about the relationship between policy and practice and about practice itself, is essential. Second, creating conditions that provoke thinking and in particular critical thinking is also essential. This means reading – not just wading through piles of official documents but reading a wide-ranging selection of articles and books; it means opportunities to discuss with colleagues and others, including outsiders who can bring new perspectives and questions (akin, perhaps, to the *pedagogistas* in the early childhood services in Reggio Emilia, Italy); and it means opportunities to visit other services and practitioners, both locally and further afield.

A third condition is providing tools for thinking about and analysing change. If something is to change, then it is important to understand better what the hindrances to change are and to have a theory about how these might be overcome to enable something different and better to be constructed. In this respect, the work in Sweden that has attempted to understand the different cultures and traditions of pre-school and school, so as to find ways of working with and beyond these differences, seems an important example. More generally, recognising that particular policies, provisions and practices are inscribed with particular theories, understandings (of children, learning, care, and so on) and principles seems far from 'merely' academic, but rather important for constructing effective processes of change. This leads us to think, for example, that social constructionist theory about childhood could be further developed into a useful analytical tool for policy making and practice development, as well as contributing further to cross-national research.

A fourth condition supported by our three case studies involves the existence of 'strategies of change' and the significance of key politicians at national and local levels to commit to change.

We chose the title for this book – *A New Deal for children?* – as a somewhat playful reference to the UK government's preoccupation with change as 'modernisation' and with the virtue of all things new. But it does raise an important question: whether the reforms in England, Scotland and Sweden can be said to constitute a significant change for the better in policy towards and for children. The answer is not straightforward, not least because so much is still uncertain about the consequences of reform. Furthermore, at one level it is clear that policies in all three countries have not made a clear break with the past and are in many aspects anything but new. Indeed, we have emphasised the strong continuities in all three countries, which are inevitable if it is accepted that certain mindsets, like those relating to welfare regimes, are deeply embedded in national psyches and are well able to survive changes of government.

There is no new deal if that means a sudden and complete break with the past. But the title of the book is more justified if we treat a new deal as in a game of cards, with children being dealt a new hand – not a totally new set of cards but a new combination, opening up more new possibilities than the previous hand. In Sweden, the new deal consists of some important changes to the institutionalisation that most Swedish children experience for much of their childhoods. There are some structural changes, such as the transfer of six year olds into school and the emergence of whole-day schools, which took place in the 1990s, followed by structural changes in the workforce, starting in the 2000s. And these are taking place within a wider conceptual landscape that holds out the prospect of a new educational system, fully embracing pre-schools and free-time services.

In England and Scotland, the New Deal has not, so far at least, been so apparent in new programmes and initiatives, which can be seen as complementing a modest programme of nursery education and as the latest and largest production in a long-running and regularly revised drama of pinning hopes on national redemption through children that we have discussed elsewhere (Moss and Petrie, 2002). The touchstone of a future New Deal will be the willingness of government to extend targeted programmes to a wider population. There are glimmerings here, for example, the general 'rolling out' of the Scottish New Community Schools initiative and the Chancellor's reference in the 2003 pre-budget statement to his goal of a Children's Centre for every community (Brown, 2003b): time will be the judge of whether these are harbingers of a New Deal.

This is to look forward. But looking back over the past few years, what may turn out to have been the most significant for the future are the signs of a new relationship to children, albeit still ambivalent: a continuing strong tendency to dwell on the 'child in need', but a recognition of the 'universal child' in the sense of being a citizen and bearer of rights. The long default position of the child located in the private sphere of the family is being disturbed by some glimmerings of the 'public child', replete with voice, rights and citizenship. While much 'joined-upnesss' is about bringing stronger, more effective means to bear on the 'poor child', it may be that the 1990s comes to be recognised as the moment when government came to recognise and engage with children as a constituency.

References

Abrahamson, P. (2002) 'Quo vadis? The future of the Nordic welfare state', *Nordic Journal of Social Work*, vol 22, no 3B, pp 6-13.

Accounts Commission (2002) *Performance indicators 1999/2000: Education services*, Edinburgh: Accounts Commission.

Audit Scotland (2001) *A good start: Commissioning pre-school education*, Edinburgh: Accounts Commission.

Baker, B. (1998) '"Childhood" in the emergence and spread of the US public school', in T. Popkewitz and M. Brennan (eds) *Foucault's challenge: Discourse, knowledge and power in education*, New York, NY: Teachers College Press, pp 117-39.

Berger, P. and Luckman, T. (1966) *The social construction of reality*, New York, NY: Doubleday.

Bertram, T. and Pascal, C. (2002) 'Early years education: an international perspective' (available at www.inca.org.uk).

Blaiklock, A.J., Kiro, C.A., Belgrave, M., Low, W., Davenport, E. and Hassall, I.B. (2002) *When the invisible hand rocks the cradle: New Zealand children in a time of change*, Innocenti Working Papers, No 93, Florence: UNICEF.

Blake Stevenson (2000) *Consultancy on support to childcare partnerships*, Edinburgh: Scottish Executive.

Bloomer, K. (2001) 'Regulation of Care Act', *Children in Scotland*, Edinburgh: Children in Scotland, July, pp 7-10.

Bradley, M. (1982) *The coordination of services for children under five*, Windsor: NFER-Nelson.

Bradshaw, J. (ed) (2002) *The well-being of children in the UK*, London: Save the Children.

Bradshaw, J., Kennedy, S., Kilkey, M., Hutton, S., Corden, A., Eardley, T., Holmes, H. and Neale, J. (1996) *Policy and the employment of lone parents in 20 countries*, York: Social Policy Research Unit, University of York.

Brannen, J. and Moss, P. (1998) 'The polarisation and intensification of parental employment in Britain: consequences for children, families and the community', *Community, Work and Family*, vol 1, no 3, pp 229-47.

Brewer, M., Goodman, A. and Shephard, A. (2003) *How has child poverty changed under the Labour government? An update*, Briefing Note No 32, London: Institute for Fiscal Studies.

Broberg, A. and Hwang, P. (1991) 'Day care for young children in Sweden', in E. Melhuish and P. Moss (eds) *Day care for young children: International perspectives*, London: Routledge.

Brown, G. (2003a) 'A modern agenda for prosperity and social reform', Speech given by the Chancellor of the Exchequer to the Social Market Foundation, 3 February (available at www.hm-treasury.gov.uk).

Brown, G. (2003b) 'Pre-budget report 2003' (available at www.hm-treasury.gov.uk).

Brown, G. (2004) 'Budget statement' (available at www.hm-treasury.gov.uk).

Bryden, J. (2003) Presentation given at 'On the move' conference, Nairn, 29 April, organised by Children in Scotland.

Cabinet Office Strategy Unit (2002) *Delivering for children and families: Inter-departmental childcare review*, London: Cabinet Office Strategy Unit.

Candappa, M. (ed) (1996) *Policy into practice: Day care services for children under eight*, London: The Stationery Office.

Central Advisory Council for Education (England) (1967) *Children and their primary schools* (Plowden Report), London: HMSO.

Children in Scotland (1999) *Manifesto for Scotland's children, young people and families: What the parties say*, Edinburgh: Children in Scotland.

Children in Scotland (2003) 'Out of the box', press release, 28 May.

Children in Scotland/Scottish Council Foundation (1999) *Children, families and learning: A new agenda for education*, Edinburgh: Scottish Council Foundation.

Cohen, B. (1990) *Caring for children: The 1990 report for the European Commission's childcare network on childcare services and policy in the UK*, London: Family Policy Studies Centre.

Cohen, B. (1998) *Children's services: Time for a fresh approach?*, Edinburgh: Scottish Local Government Information Unit.

Cohen, B. (2002) *Children in Europe, focus on ... Scotland*, Edinburgh: Children in Scotland.

Cohen, B. (2003) 'Scotland's children and the new parliament', *Children and Society*, vol 17, pp 236-46.

Cohen, B. and Hagan, U. (eds) (1997) *Children's services: Shaping up for the millennium*, Edinburgh: The Stationery Office.

Colley, L. (2002) *Captives: Britain, empire and the world*, London: Jonathan Cape.

Cunningham-Burley, S., Jamieson, L., Morton, S., Adam, R. and McFarlane, V. (2002) *Sure Start Scotland mapping exercise: Report to the Edinburgh Scottish Executive*, Edinburgh: Centre for Research on Families and Relationships.

CYPU (Children and Young People's Unit) (2001) 'Learning to listen: care principles for the involvement of children and young people' (available at www.cyou.gov.uk).

Dahlberg, G. (1997) 'Barnet och pedagogen som medkonstruktorer av kultur och kunskap' ['The child and the pedagogue as co-constructors of culture and knowledge'], *Roster om den svenska barnomsorgen* [*Voices about Swedish child care*], SoS Report, Stockholm: Socialstyrelsen.

Dahlberg, G. and Lenz Taguchi, H. (1994) *Förskola och skola – om två skilda traditioner och om visionem om en mötesplats* [*Preschool and school – two different traditions and a vision of an encounter*], Stockholm: HLS Förlag.

Dahlberg, G., Moss, P. and Pence, A. (1999) *Beyond quality in early childhood education and care: Postmodern perspectives*, London: Routledge Falmer.

Daycare Trust (2003) *Annual costs of childcare survey*, London: Daycare Trust.

DES (Department of Education and Science) (1972) *Education: A framework for expansion*, London: HMSO.

Deven, F. and Moss, P. (2002) 'Leave arrangements for parents: overview and future outlook', *Community, Work & Family*, vol 5, no 3, pp 237-55.

Devine, T.M. (1999) *The Scottish nation 1700–2000*, London: Penguin Books.

DfEE (Department for Education and Employment) (1998) *Meeting the childcare challenge*, London: The Stationery Office.

DfES (Department for Education and Skills) (2001) *Children's day care facilities at 31 March*, London: DfES.

DfES (2002) *Schools: Achieving success*, London: DfES.

DfES (2003a) *Every child matters*, Cm 5860, London: The Stationery Office.

DfES (2003b) 'Margaret Hodge appointed Minister of State for Children and reforms for children's services', press release, 13 June.

Dobrowolsky, A. (2002) 'Rhetoric versus reality: the figure of the child and New Labour's strategic "social investment state"', *Studies in Political Economy*, Issue 69, pp 43-73.

DoH (Department of Health) (1991) *The Children Act 1989 guidance and regulations: Volume 2, family support, day care and educational provision for young children*, London: HMSO.

DoH (1997) *Children's Day care facilities at 31 March*, London: DoH.

DoH and DfES (2003) *Children's trusts: Interdepartmental guide*, London: DfES.

Duffield, M. (2002) 'Trends in female employment 2002', *Labour Market Trends*, vol 110, no 11, pp 605-16.

Escobeda, A., Fernandez, E., Moreno, D. and Moss, P. (2002) 'Surveying demand, supply and use of care: consolidated report for care work in Europe study' (available at http://144.82.35.228/carework/uk/index.htm).

Esping-Andersen, G. (1999) *Social foundations of postindustrial economies*, Oxford: Oxford University Press.

Esping-Andersen, G., Gallie, D., Hemerijk, A. and Myles, J. (2001) *A new welfare architecture for Europe: Report submitted to the Belgian presidency of the European Union*, September.

European Commission Childcare Network (1996) *A review of services for young children, 1990-1995*, Brussels: European Commission Equal Opportunities Unit.

European Council of Ministers Recommendation on Child Care (1992) Brussels.

Eurostat (Statistical Office of the European Communities) (2002) *The social situation in the European Union 2002*, Annex II, I, Luxembourg: Office for Official Publications of the European Communities.

Evans, M. (2003a) 'All together', *Nursery World*, 15 May, pp 10-11.

Evans, M. (2003b) 'Put in the shade', *Nursery World*, 10 April, pp 10-11.

Evans, M. (2003c) 'Paying off?', *Nursery World*, 13 November, pp 10-11.

Fawcett, B., Featherstone, B. and Goddard, J. (2003) 'From the womb to the workplace: child welfare under New Labour', Paper presented to the annual conference of the Social Policy Association, University of Teesside, Middlesbrough, 15 July.

Fendler, L. (2001) 'Educating flexible souls', in K. Hultqvist and G. Dahlberg (eds) *Governing the child in the new millennium*, London: Routledge Falmer.

Flising, B. (2003) Personal communication, University of Göteborg.

Flising, L. (2002) 'Material from Sweden to the project on school inclusion: an international review', Unpublished report prepared for Thomas Coram Research Unit, University of London.

Fritzell, J. (1999) 'Still different? Income distribution in the Nordic countries in a European comparison', in M. Kautto, J. Fritzell, B. Hvinden, J. Kvist and H. Uusitalo (eds) *Nordic welfare states in the European context*, London: Routledge.

Galbraith, S. (1998) 'Local authorities and early years services', paper presented to a Children in Scotland conference, Edinburgh, January,

Gergen, K. and Gergen, M. (1991) 'Towards reflexive methodologies', in F. Steier (ed) *Research and reflexivity*, London: Sage Publications.

Glass, N. (1999) 'Sure Start: the development of an early intervention programme for young children in the United Kingdom', *Children & Society*, vol 13, no 4, pp 257-64.

Gray, J. (1998) *False dawn: The delusions of global capitalism*, London: Granta Books.

GROS (General Registrar Office for Scotland) (2001) *Revised mid-year estimates for 1982-90 and 1990-2000 for all of Scotland's under 5's*, Edinburgh: GROS.

Gunnarsson, L., Korpi, B.M. and Nordenstam, U. (1999) *Early childhood education and care in Sweden: Background report prepared for the OECD thematic review*, Stockholm: Swedish Ministry of Education and Science.

Haas, L. and Hwang, P. (1999) 'Parental leave in Sweden', in P. Moss and F. Deven (eds) *Parental leave: progress or pitfall?*, The Hague and Brussels: NIDI CBGS Publications, pp 45-68.

Hall, D.M.B. (2003) *Health for all children*, Oxford: Oxford Medical Publications.

Harvey, D. (1989) *The condition of postmodernity*, Oxford: Blackwell.

HMIE (Her Majesty's Inspectorate of Education in Scotland) (2002) *Standards and quality in Scottish pre-school education 1997–2001*, Edinburgh: The Stationery Office.

HM Inspectors of Schools in Scotland (1994) *The education of children under five in Scotland*, Edinburgh: Scottish Office Education Department.

HM Inspectors of Schools in Scotland (1995) *Performance indicators and self-evaluation for pre-school centres*, Edinburgh: Scottish Office Education and Industry Department.

HM Inspectors of Schools in Scotland (1997) *Curriculum framework for children in their pre-school year*, Edinburgh: Scottish Office Education and Industry Department.

HM Treasury (2000) *Budget 2000: Prudent for a purpose, working for a stronger and fairer Britain*, London: The Stationery Office.

Hughes, C., Hamilton, D. and Tisdall, E. (2001) *Children's rights audit 2000-2001: An overview of Scottish Executive and parliamentary activity in relation to children and young people*, Edinburgh: Children in Scotland/UNICEF.

Inland Revenue (2003a) 'Working Families Tax Credit statistics: quarterly enquiry, United Kingdom', August (available at www.inlandrevenue.gov.uk).

Inland Revenue (2003b) 'Working Families Tax Credit statistics: quarterly enquiry, United Kingdom', October (available at www.inlandrevenue.gov.uk/stats/index.htm).

Jackson, P. (2003) 'HALL4: why we should all know what it means', Children in Scotland magazine article, September, p 6.

Jenks, C. (1982) The sociology of childhood: Essential readings, London: Batsford Academic.

Kagan, S. (1997) 'Support systems for children, families and schools in inner-city situations', Education and Urban Society, vol 29, no 3, pp 277-95.

Kendall, L. and Harker, L. (2002) 'A vision for social care', in L. Kendall and L. Harker (eds) From welfare to wellbeing: The future of social care, London: Institute for Public Policy Research.

King, M. (1997) A better world for children: Explorations in morality and authority, London: Routledge.

Kinney, L. (2002) 'Childcare Partnerships', Children in Scotland, April.

Kommittén Välfärdsbokslut (2000) Two of a kind? Economic crisis, policy responses and welfare during the 1990s in Sweden and Finland (SOU 2000, p 83), Stockholm: Socialdepartementet.

Konrad, E. L. (1996) 'A multidimensional framework for conceptualising human services integration initiatives', in J.M. Marquand and E.L. Konrad (eds) Evaluating initiatives to integrate human services, San Francisco, CA: Jossey-Bass, pp 5-19.

Kristoffersson, M. (1998) Föräldrasamverkan "Lokala styrelser" – är det en bra modell för inflytande?, Finland: Nordisk förening för Pedagogisk Forskning i Lathi.

Kvist, J. (2002) 'Is the Nordic welfare model viable?', Nordic Journal of Social Work, vol 22, no 3B, pp 20-30.

Labour Party (1997) Early excellence: A head start for every child, London: Labour Party.

Laing and Buisson (2003) Children's nurseries: UK market sector report 2003, London: Laing and Buisson.

Lenz Taguchi, H. and Munkammer, I. (2003) Consolidating governmental early childhood education and care services under the Ministry of Education and Care: A Swedish case study, UNESCO Early Childhood and Family Policy Series No 6 (available at www.unesco.org).

Lidholt, B. (1999) Adjustment, fight and escape: How pre-school staff cope with effects of financial cutbacks and other changes, Uppsala: Acta Universitatis Upsaliensis.

Lister, R. (2003) 'Investing in the citizens-workers of the future: transformations in citizenship and the state under New Labour', *Social Policy and Administration*, vol 37, no 5, pp 427-43.

Luxembourg Income Study (2000a) 'Relative poverty rates for the total population, children and the elderly' (available at www.lisproject.org/keyfigures/povertytable.htm).

Luxembourg Income Study (2000b) 'Poverty rates for children by family type' (available at www.lisproject.org/keyfigures/povertytable.htm)

Luxembourg Income Study (2000c) 'Income inequality measures' (available at www.lisproject.org/keyfigures/povertytable.htm).

Luxembourg Income Study (2000d) 'Distribution of children living in different income households' (available at www.lisproject.org/keyfigures/povertytable.htm).

McCrone, G. (2001) *A teaching profession for the 21st century: Volume 1 report*, Edinburgh: Scottish Executive.

Malaguzzi, L. (1993) 'For an education based on relationships', *Young Children*, November, pp 9-13

Martin, C., Wallace, J. and Bell, A. (2003) *Insight 10: Awards in early education, childcare and playwork*, Edinburgh: Scottish Executive.

Marx, I. (1999) 'Low pay and poverty in OECD countries', *Employment Audit*, vol 10, pp 17-21.

Maturana, H. (1991) 'Science and daily life: the ontology of scientific explanations', F. Steier (ed) *Research and reflexivity*, London: Sage Publications.

Meade, A. and Podmore, V. (2001) 'Early childhood education policy coordination under the auspices of the Department/Ministry of Education: a case study of New Zealand' (available at www.unesco.org).

Melaville, A.I. and Blank, M.J. (1999) 'Trends and lessons in school-community initiatives', Paper delivered at national invitational conference on 'Improving Results for Children and Families by Connecting Collaborative Services with School Reform Efforts', Laboratory for Student Success, Temple University Center for Research in Human Development and Education, Washington DC.

Mercer, A. (2003) 'School transition under scrutiny', *Nursery World*, 5 June, pp 4-5.

Milburn, A. (2002) Speech to the Annual Social Services Conference, Cardiff, 16 October (available at www.doh.gov.uk)

Mooney, A., Knight, A., Moss, P. and Owen, C. (2001) *Who cares? Childminding in the 1990s*, London: Family Policy Studies Centre, for the Joseph Rowntree Foundation.

Moss, P. (2001) 'Renewed hopes and lost opportunities: early childhood in the early years of the Labour government', in M. Fielding (ed) *Taking education really seriously: Four years hard labour*, London: Routledge Falmer.

Moss, P. (2002) 'Getting beyond childcare: reflections on recent policy and future possibilities', in J. Brannen and P. Moss (eds) *Rethinking children's care*, Buckingham: Open University Press, pp 25-43.

Moss, P. and Cameron, C. (2002) 'Care work and the care workforce: report on stage one and state of the art review' (available from the Carework in Europe website at www.ioe.ac.uk/tcru/carework.htm).

Moss, P. and Deven, F. (eds) (1999) *Parental leave: Progress or pitfall?*, The Hague and Brussels: NIDI CBGS Publications.

Moss, P. and Petrie, P. (1998) *Children's services: Time for a new approach*, London: Institute of Education, University of London.

Moss, P. and Petrie, P. (2002) *From children's services to children's spaces*, London: Taylor and Francis.

Moss, P., Dillon, J. and Statham, J. (2000) 'The "child in need" and the "rich child": discourses, constructions and practice', *Critical Social Policy*, vol 20, no 2, pp 233-54.

Moss, P., Petrie, P. and Poland, G. (1999) *Rethinking school: Some international perspectives*, Leicester: Youth Work Press, for the Joseph Rowntree Foundation.

National Audit Office (2004) *Early years: Progress in developing high quality childcare and early education accessible to all*, London: The Stationery Office.

New Zealand Ministry of Education (2002) *Pathways to the future: A 10-year strategic plan for early childhood education*, Wellington: New Zealand Ministry of Education.

Nursery Market News (2003) 'Just learning acquisition takes consolidation to new levels', *Nursery Market News*, vol 2, no 2, pp 205-6.

OECD (Organisation for Economic Co-operation and Development) (2001) *Starting strong*, Paris: OECD.

OECD (2002) *Revenue statistics, 1965-2001*, Paris: OECD.

OECD (2003) *OECD in figures* (2003 edn), Paris: OECD.

ONS (Office for National Statistics) (2002) 'Tables', *Population Trends*, no 110, pp 42-70.

ONS (2003a) *Provision for children under five years of age in England January 2003 (provisional)*, London: DfES.

ONS (2003b) *Social trends No 33 (2003 edition)*, London: The Stationery Office.

Palmer, G., North, J., Carr, J. and Kenway, P. (2003) *Monitoring poverty and social exclusion 2003*, York: Joseph Rowntree Foundation.

Penn, H. (2002) *Children in Scotland April 2002*, Edinburgh: Children in Scotland.

Petrie, P. (1994) *Play and care out of school*, London: HMSO.

Petrie, P. (2002) 'Social pedagogy: an historical account of care and education as social control', in J. Brannen and P. Moss (eds) *Rethinking children's care*, Buckingham: Open University Press, pp 61-79.

Popkewitz, T. (1998) *Struggling for the soul: The politics of schooling and the construction of the teacher*, New York, NY: Teachers College Press.

Prout, A. (2000) 'Children's participation: control and self-realisation in British late modernity', *Children & Society*, vol 14, pp 304-15.

Prout, A. and James, A. (1997) 'A new paradigm for the sociology of childhood', in A. James and A. Prout (eds) *Constructing and deconstructing childhood: Contemporary issues in the sociological study of childhood*, London: Falmer Books.

QCA (Qualifications and Curriculum Authority) (2000) *Curriculum guidance for the Foundation Stage*, London: QCA and DfEE.

Rendall, M. and Smallwood, S. (2003) 'Higher qualifications, first-birth timing and further childbearing in England and Wales', *Population Trends*, no 111, pp 18-26.

Rinaldi, C. (1999) Paper given to a British study tour to Reggio Emilia, April.

Ritchey, E. (1998) *Föräldrar – är det nåt att ha?*, Stockholm: Skorlverket.

Rose, N. (1999) *Powers of freedom: Reframing political thought*, Cambridge: Cambridge University Press.

Ryan, B. (2003) 'Service integration: a policy paradox', *Children's Issues*, vol 7, no 2, pp 36-42.

Ryan, B., Robinson, R., Forsyth, A., Lero, D., Belcher, J., Eaton, F., Hall, D., Nagy, P., Normore, A., O'Connor, P. and Smith, D. (2002) *Evaluation of the healthy babies, healthy children program*, Toronto: Ministry of Health and Long-Term Care.

Sammons, P., Power, S., Elliot, K., Robertson, P., Campbell, C. and Whitty, G. (2002) *Interchange 76, National evaluation of the New Community Schools pilot programme in Scotland, Phase 1*, Edinburgh: Scottish Executive.

Sammons, P., Power, S., Elliot, K., Robertson, P., Campbell, C. and Whitty, G. (2003) *New Community Schools in Scotland final report: National evaluation of the pilot phase*, London: Institute of Education, University of London.

Schofield, J. (2001) 'Swedes skate ahead', *Guardian* (Online section), 22 March.

Scotland Office (2002) *Devolution Guidance Notes: DGN3*, London: HMSO.

Scottish Consultative Council on the Curriculum (1999) *A Curriculum Framework for Children 3 – 5*, Edinburgh: Scottish Office.

Scottish Executive (2000) *The child at the centre: Self-evaluation in the early years*, Edinburgh: Scottish Executive.

Scottish Executive (2001a) *For Scotland's children: Better integrated children's services*, Edinburgh: Scottish Executive.

Scottish Executive (2001b) *Planning for children's services. Annex D Sure Start Scotland Bulletin 1*, Edinburgh: Scottish Executive.

Scottish Executive (2001c) *Sure Start Scotland programme*, Edinburgh: The Stationery Office.

Scottish Executive (2001d) 'We cannot fail our children, say Ministers', press release, October, Edinburgh: Scottish Executive.

Scottish Executive (2002a) *National care standards: Early education and childcare up to the age of 16*, Edinburgh: Scottish Executive.

Scottish Executive (2002b) *The National Debate on Education: Emerging views*, Edinburgh: Scottish Executive.

Scottish Executive (2003a) *A partnership for a better Scotland*, Edinburgh: Scottish Executive.

Scottish Executive (2003b) *Integrated strategy for the early years*, Edinburgh: Scottish Executive.

Scottish Executive (2003c) *Educating for excellence: The Executive's response to the national debate*, Edinburgh: Scottish Executive.

Scottish Executive (2003d) *Response to Petition PE 523 calling for the Scottish Executive to initiate an inquiry into early years education and childcare: Meeting the Minister,* Edinburgh: Children in Scotland, July.

Scottish Executive (2003e) *Schools out: Framework for the development of out of school care*, Edinburgh: Scottish Executive.

Scottish Executive (2003f) *The 2003 pre-school and daycare census,* July.

Scottish Office (1991) *Guidance to local authorities on the Children Act 1989*, Edinburgh: Scottish Office.

Scottish Office (1996) *Statistical bulletin – Social work series services for children 1995*, Edinburgh: Scottish Office.

Scottish Office (1998a) *Report on the Scottish Office seminar for HM Government's cross-departmental review on provision for young children*, Edinburgh: Children in Scotland/Scottish Office.

Scottish Office (1998b) 'New community schools: the prospectus', Edinburgh: Scottish Office (www.scotland.gov.uk/library/documents-w3).

Scottish Office (1998c) *Meeting the childcare challenge: A childcare strategy for Scotland*, Edinburgh: The Stationery Office.

Seenan, G. (2003) 'Scotland launches drive to draw in foreign workers', *The Guardian*, 26 February.

Sennett, R. (1998) *The corrosion of character: The personal consequences of work in the new capitalism*, London: Norton Books.

Sevenhuijsen, S. (2002) 'A third way? Moralities, ethics and families: an approach through the ethic of care', in A. Carling, S. Duncan and R. Edwards (eds) *Analysing families: Morality and rationality in policy and practice*, London: Routledge.

Shaw, C. (2003) 'Interim 2001-based national population projections for the United Kingdom and its constituent countries', *Population Trends*, no 111, pp 7-17.

Shephard, A. (2003) *Inequality under the Labour government? An update*, Briefing Note No 33, London: Institute for Fiscal Studies.

Skinner, A. (2001) 'Regulation of Care Act', *Children in Scotland*, Edinburgh: Children in Scotland, July.

Skolverket (2000) 'Barns omsorg', Rapport no 203, Stockholm: Skolverket.

Skolverket (2001a) nr 201: *Att bygga en ny skolform för 6-åringarna – Om integrationen förskoleklass, grundskola och fritidshem*, Stockholm: Skolverket.

Skolverket (2001b) Report No 192, *Descriptive data on childcare and school in Sweden*, Stockholm: Skolverket.

Skolverket (2003) nr 229: *Barnomsorg, skola, vuxenutbildning*, Del 1, 2003, Organisation – Personal – Resultat, Stockholm: Skolverket.

Socialstyrelsen (1997) *Röster om den svenska barnomsorgen*, En antologi SoS-rapport, Stockholm: SOS.

SOU (1974: 53) *Skolans arbetsmiljö*, Stockholm: Utbildnings Departementet.

SOU (1995) *Föräldrar i självförvaltande skolor Delbetänkande av Skolkommittén*, Stockholm: Allmänna Förlaget.

Statham, J., Dillon, J. and Moss, P. (2001) *Placed and paid for: Supporting families through sponsored day care*, London: The Stationery Office.

Stewart, G. (1999) 'The new children and young people's group', *Children in Scotland*, July, Edinburgh: Children in Scotland.

Sure Start Unit (2003a) *Children's centres – developing integrated services for young children and their families: Start up guidance*, London: Sure Start Unit.

Sure Start Unit (2003b) *Birth to three matters: A framework to support children in their earliest days*, London: DfES.

Sutherland, H., Sefton, T. and Piachaud, D. (2003) *Progress on poverty, 1997 to 2003/4: Findings*, York: Joseph Rowntree Foundation.

Swedish Children's Ombudsman (2001) *Facts on children and youth*, Stockholm: Children's Ombudsman.

Swedish Ministry of Education and Science (1994) *Läroplan för det obligatoriska skolväsendet, förskoleklassen och fritidshemmet, Lpfö94 [Curriculum for the compulsory school, pre-school class and free-time services]*, Stockholm: Swedish Ministry of Education and Science.

Swedish Ministry of Education and Science (1998) *Läroplan för förskolan, Lpfö98 [Curriculum for pre-school]*, Stockholm: Swedish Ministry of Education and Science, p 1.

Swedish Ministry of Education and Science (2000) 'Maximum fees in universal pre-school', Factsheet v00.017, May 2000, Stockholm: Swedish Ministry of Education and Science, p 1.

Tisdall, E.K.M. (1997) *The Children (Scotland) Act 1995: Developing policy and law for Scotland's children*, Edinburgh: The Stationery Office.

Tweed, J. (2003) 'Foundation post delights sector', *Nursery World*, 25 September, p 4.

UNICEF (2000) *A league table of child poverty in rich countries*, Innocenti Report Card Issue No 1 (available at www.unicef-icdc.org).

United Nations Development Programme (2003) 'Human Development Report 2003' (available at www.undp.org).

University of Gothenburg (2001) *Lararprogrammet 120-220 paang*, Gothenburg.

Vanderwoerd, J. (1996) *Service provider involvement report: Integrating agencies into the Onward Willow Better Beginnings, Better Futures project*, Kingston, Ontario: Better Beginnings, Better Future Research Coordination Unit, Queens University.

Vegeris, S. and Perry, J. (2003) *Families and children 2001: Living standards and the children)* (research summary), London: DWP.

Wang, M.C., Haertel, G.D. and Walberg, H.J. (1998) *The effectiveness of collaborative school-linked services* (available at www.temple.edu/LSS, Laboratory for Student Success).

Whitty, G., Power, S. and Halperin, D. (1998) *Devolution and choice in education*, Buckingham: Open University Press.

Wilkinson, E. (2003) *Early childhood education: The new agenda*, Policy and Practice in Education No 6, Edinburgh: Dunedin Academic Press.

Woodland, S., Miller, M. and Tipping, S. (2002) *Repeat study of parents' demand for childcare*, Research Report 348, London: DfES.

Wragg, T. (2003) 'Wise words', *Guardian Education*, 4 March, p 5.

Fieldwork

For each country, fieldwork was conducted at national level and in three local authorities, selected on the basis of their varied characteristics.

For all three countries, documentation was collected at the national level and the local level.

The main informants are listed below. Where relevant, the researchers had guided visits to the services in which the main informants were based; they also took the opportunity to engage in conversations with other members of staff in these services.

England

National fieldwork 2001-02

Twenty-four interviews were conducted with 33 informants (nine interviews were with two or three informants). Eight interviews were with informants in government departments (DfES, DoH, DCMS, HM Treasury including a senior politician); two with informants in public bodies (Ofsted and QCA); two with trade unions (NUT and UNISON); six with voluntary organisations; and six with individual researchers and other experts.

Local case study 1, main informants

Five local authority administrators, including the lead officer on the EYDCP, and one development worker, one head of out-of-school care service, two nursery school head teachers, one head teacher of primary school, one school-based community worker, one head teacher of a middle school, one proprietor of a children's centre (13 main informants).

Local case study 2, main informants

Five local government administrators and three development workers, one head of a local authority nursery school, one head of an out-of-school club, two head teachers of primary schools, with nursery classes and out-of-school services, one deputy head of a secondary school, one out-of-school leader (14 main informants).

Local case study 3, main informants

Eight local authority administrators and development officers, the council leader, the manager of an Early Excellence Centre, one nursery school head teacher, three primary head teachers and one acting head (15 informants).

Sweden

National fieldwork 2002

Fifteen interviews were conducted with 21 informants. Four interviews involved two or three informants. Four interviews were with civil servants or advisers based in government agencies, one with trade union officials, one with a local government association and nine with educationists (21 informants).

Local case study 1, main informants

Two administrators, two practitioners working across the local authority, three pre-school teachers, 12 compulsory teachers, one free-time pedagogue (lower school), one *rektor* in charge of a cluster of services (21 main informants).

Local case study 2, main informants

Four local authority administrators, one *rektor* of a special school, one *rektor* of a cluster of schools, one vice *rektor* of a school incorporating both pre-school and the pre-school class, one vice *rektor* and three class teachers from a school for 13- to 16-year-olds; two vice *rektors* from schools for children from six to 12 years. Three pre-school teachers, three leisure pedagogues, eight class teachers from schools for children from six to 13 years, one school nurse and six members of both the junior and senior schools pupil councils (including the chair of the senior schools council) (34 main informants).

Local case study 3, main informants

Five local authority administrators and development workers; one deputy *rektor* of a school for children aged six to 16, with two associated pre-schools, one deputy *rektor* of a school for 13- to 16-year-olds, one free-time pedagogue, one pre-school class teacher, one teacher of seven-year-olds and three secondary school teachers (13 main informants).

Scotland

National fieldwork 2001-02

At national level, 18 interviews were conducted with 25 informants (five interviews were with two or more informants) and included representatives of the Scottish Executive Education Department (three), Her Majesty's Inspectorate of Education (four) and the Social Work Inspectorate (one), four representatives of local government, seven representatives from the voluntary sector, one representative of the private childcare sector, two academics, one representative of the teachers' union, one representative of the Scottish Executive Social Inclusion Department and one senior politician.

Local case study 1, main informants

Three local authority administrators and development workers, one primary school head teacher, one teacher responsible for pupil support, one social care worker, one learning support auxiliary, one head teacher and one integration manager of a New Community Secondary school, one private day nursery proprietor, four staff of a youth project service and one voluntary sector development worker (15 main informants).

Local case study 2, main informants

Three local authority administrators and development workers; one senior play worker and one play worker in an out-of-school care service, one head teacher of a primary school, the deputy rector of a secondary school and the manager of a pre-school nursery (eight main informants).

Local case study 3, main informants

Three local authority workers, one head teacher and one deputy head teacher of a primary school, one secondary head teacher, one coordinator of an out-of-school service, one coordinator and two staff at a nursery and out-of-school service (10 main informants).

Index

Page numbers in *italics* refer to tables or case studies.

Also available from The Policy Press

Learning for life
The foundations for lifelong learning

David H. Hargreaves

Paperback £14.99 (US$25.00) ISBN 1 86134 597 6
234 x156mm 128 pages May 2004

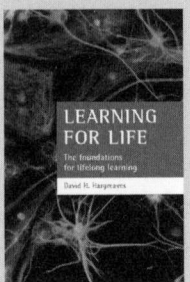

To order further copies of this publication or any other Policy Press title please contact:

In the UK and Europe:
Marston Book Services, PO Box 269, Abingdon, Oxon, OX14 4YN, UK
Tel: +44 (0)1235 465500, Fax: +44 (0)1235 465556,
Email: direct.orders@marston.co.uk

In the USA and Canada:
ISBS, 920 NE 58th Street, Suite 300, Portland, OR 97213-3786, USA
Tel: +1 800 944 6190 (toll free), Fax: +1 503 280 8832,
Email: info@isbs.com

In Australia and New Zealand:
DA Information Services, 648 Whitehorse Road, Mitcham, Victoria 3132, Australia
Tel: +61 (3) 9210 7777, Fax: +61 (3) 9210 7788,
E-mail: service@dadirect.com.au

Further information about all of our titles can be also be found on our website:

www.policypress.org.uk